MY VICTORY AGAINST VITILIGO

A Successful Story & a Practical Guide to Treatment

XICHAO MO

MY VICTORY AGAINST VITILIGO

COPYRIGHT ©2014 BY XICHAO MO

PACLINX PUBLISHING

www.paclinx.com

ISBN-13: 978-0-615-96100-2
ISBN-10:   0-615-96100-2

FIRST EDITION

This book is dedicated to the people who are affected by vitiligo.

CONTENTS

Acknowledgements

Sincere thanks to my wife, daughter, and son for their loyal support during my battle against vitiligo, and for their valuable inputs on this book.

Special thanks to my mom and dad, as well as other beloved family members and friends, for the information and assistance they have warmly provided.

I am also very grateful to the people who shared their successful stories on the internet. These people and their stories provided me with the much-needed strength and inspiration at a critical time, and were the key to my successful recovery.

Disclaimer

The purpose of this book is to share experiences and information on vitiligo treatment. It is also intended to encourage people to take a positive outlook on the situation and explore their best options in the journey to a complete recovery.

All the information referenced in this book regarding medicines and medical studies can be found from credible sources in the public domain. Readers are encouraged to check the information provided before making any treatment decisions or lifestyle changes.

The author evaluated the risks of various treatments and made personal decisions to use certain combination of therapies, which might not be safe or effective for other individuals who are affected by vitiligo. Therefore, his experiences, although true and successful, shall not be considered as a recommendation or endorsement for certain treatments.

Please be further advised that the author of this book is NOT a physician and the information in this book SHALL NOT be deemed as medical advice. The author is not responsible for the actions taken as a result from reading this book. Readers shall consult their physicians for medical advice and directions on vitiligo treatments.

Introduction

Many of the people who are affected by vitiligo have been told by their dermatologists that there was no cure for this condition, and there was not much that could be done.

Five years ago, I was also given the same pessimistic verdicts by a few dermatologists. As the condition got worse, I refused to believe that my best option was to do nothing. From my experience as an engineer, I know the world is changing rapidly and it is dangerous to make assumptions without keeping up with the latest development. So I started collecting information and tried to find solutions.

As I found out, these verdicts are wrong!

While it is true that the causes of vitiligo are not yet fully understood by the medical community and no universal cure has been found, there are plenty of effective and affordable treatments that can help. In fact, many people have proved with their experiences that vitiligo can be healed.

Some of these treatments might be expensive, but many others are very affordable to the average patients. After two years of trial and error, I finally recovered from this unpleasant condition by using some of the inexpensive and painless therapies.

This book will tell you about my personal experience and the valuable knowledge I have come across during my research. There is no single treatment that works for every patient at the time of writing, but you sure can find a solution that works best for you.

I sincerely hope that this book will bring you the hope, encouragement, inspiration, and knowledge needed to pave the road to your victory.

1. My Story

THE WHITE SPOTS

A few months after moving to a different city, I noticed a couple of faint white spots on my face. Since they were very small and would come and go, I didn't take them seriously at that time.

One year later, a small white patch slowly emerged near the inside corner of my left eyebrow. This patch was about the size of a dime and this time it wouldn't go away. A few hairs within the patch also turned white. I was alarmed and decided to see a dermatologist.

I made an appointment with dermatologist Dr. H and went to see him on a Friday afternoon. Dr. H decided a skin biopsy was necessary, so he used a needle to take some tissue off from the white patch. He then prescribed triamcinolone acetonide cream, and asked me to rub it on the white patch twice a day.

"Don't use it for more than a couple months." He told me. I later realized that the cream was a type of topical corticosteroid and could cause skin thinning.

THE VERDICT

A few weeks later, I went back for a follow-up. Dr. H delivered the bad news to me: the biopsy ruled out other infections. He believed what I had was vitiligo.

Vitiligo! It was a terrifying word for me. Nobody in my family, starting from my grandparents, had ever been affected by vitiligo, but I heard about it before and knew it was a tough condition to treat.

My first question to Dr. H was, "Is it curable?"

Dr. H answered my question very diplomatically, "In the medical field, we don't use the word cure; we prefer the word treatment. The outcome will depend on how a patient responds to the treatment." I knew right away what he was trying to say: I don't have a good solution to your problem.

Since the triamcinolone acetonide cream didn't seem to make much of a difference thus far, Dr. H prescribed another topical medication for me.

"This medicine can be quite expensive." He kindly warned me of the cost. The new medicine was the Protopic 0.1% ointment. At that time, I had no clue how popular it was in vitiligo treatment.

The Protopic ointment was indeed quite expensive. Even with a decent insurance plan, I still ended up paying over fifty dollars for a small tube. Dr. H told me to use the triamcinolone acetonide cream in the mornings and the Protopic ointment in the evenings, and that I could even experiment mixing the two together.

"Don't use them for too long," He reminded me.

I followed his instructions and used the cream and ointment for about two months. The condition was not getting better, but not worse either. With Dr. H's warning in mind, I put the medicines away.

LEAVING IT ALONE

Several months later, I visited my primary care doctor for a routine physical checkup. He noticed the white spot on my eyebrow and gave me the phone number of Dr. B, a dermatologist he knew. Because of his recommendation, I was under the impression that Dr. B was an expert in vitiligo. At that time, the white patch was getting a little bigger. I made an appointment with dermatologist Dr. B, thinking a second opinion was not a bad idea.

Dr. B took out a Wood's lamp and checked my face for a minute in the dark room. Then she said, "Yeah, I think it is vitiligo. There is no effective medication for this, so I would just suggest that you relax and leave it alone."

For a few hundred dollars, that was certainly an expensive piece of medical advice. But at the same time, I was relieved that I didn't have to take any medicines or go through surgeries. So, I happily took the advice from Dr. B: leave it alone, just relax and be hopeful that someday it would disappear.

GETTING WORSE

As time went by, the white patch on my eyebrow gradually got bigger. A year and a half after the diagnosis, several small spots slowly showed up on the left side of my nose, and eventually merged into another big patch. Now I had two big white patches on my face.

Apparently, the "leaving it alone" strategy was not working, and I got a little worried. My imagination went for a wild ride, trying to figure out what was causing the problem.

I first noticed something interesting: all the white patches on my face stayed on the left side so far; they didn't cross the center line of my face. Since I traveled south to work in the morning and drove north back home in the afternoon five days a week, I wondered if the sun, which always shined on my left side, had anything to do with the condition.

I also noticed that the white spots seemed to have something to do with the food I ate. Sometimes they got a little smaller; sometimes they got bigger even when my general health condition didn't seem to have changed.

The white spots showed up after I moved to the east coast of Florida. Was it possible that the local food and water had something to do with them?

Another issue also caught my attention. About one year before I noticed any white spot, I started experiencing periodic abdominal pain and loose bowel movements, which had come and gone throughout the following years. This was certainly an issue that warranted serious investigation. Unfortunately, I visited several doctors and none of them was able to give me a good explanation. I even had a colonoscopy procedure, but everything was normal according to the report. Could this have any connection with vitiligo?

THE HOMEMADE PSORALEN SOLUTION

I saw some home remedies on the internet and decided to give them a shot. The first remedy I decided to try was a type of topical psoralen solution because it was easy to make.

I had my cousin pick up some babchi seeds (also known as psoralea corylifolia) from an herb store. These seeds looked like black peppers from far away. I put them in a glass bottle, which was then filled up with 70% ethyl rubbing alcohol. The directions stated using 75% alcohol, however I didn't like the smell of the isopropyl alcohol sold in the drug stores. The smell of the ethyl alcohol was better but still quite unpleasant. I later switched to a type of rice liquor that contained 55% alcohol and preferred its natural aroma.

The homemade psoralen solution was ready after 10 days or so. I then separated the seeds from the solution so the concentration would not increase overtime. Psoralen solution of very high concentrations could make the skin overly sensitive to the sunlight.

I applied the solution to the white patches once a day at night using cotton swabs. In the first month, I accidentally ignored the instruction on getting 20 minutes of direct sunlight exposure after applying the solution, and didn't see any improvement.

Once I started getting sunlight exposure, the patches would turn pink after several hours, apparently because the skin was getting more photosensitive. It was working! With the pink tone, the lesions would blend in better with the surrounding healthy skin and appeared to be less noticeable. However, once the erythema faded away, the lesions only seemed to be marginally better.

The lesson I learned was that the application of the solution and the sunlight exposure must be carefully controlled. Very often, I would apply many layers of the solution on the lesions and that made the skin overly sensitive. Since the erythema wouldn't happen right away, it was easy to get overexposure from the sunlight. I could only realize the problem when the severe erythema showed up after several hours, but it was too late.

Overexposure caused the lesions to turn red or even purple. The outer skin layer would be burned and then start peeling off after a few days. Overexposure was certainly harmful. It could even cause the lesions to spread if the vitiligo was in the active stage.

In my case, this remedy appeared to work for small spots that just showed up, but was not effective for bigger ones. After a while, the white patches seemed to be stabilized, and I stopped using the psoralen solution.

THE ENVIRONMENTAL FACTORS

I have always suspected that certain environmental factors might have played a role in the development of my condition. To test this theory, I decided to get away from the city in which I live and spend some time with my parents in my hometown.

It was the winter season, the weather was humid and cold in my hometown. Near the end of the multi-week stay, I noticed two or three very faint white spots on my left cheek. They were not significant, but I was alarmed.

After I came back home, the new spots started to get lighter and bigger. Eventually, they merged with each other and my face now had several white patches and looked awful. Sensing something bad was going on, I was both frightened and depressed.

Very likely, the stay at my hometown had something to do with the new development. But what had caused it? Was it the cold weather? Was it the water? Or was it the spicy food?

I resumed the homemade psoralen treatment and accidentally got overexposed a few times. That made things even worse. The skin was burned and peeling off. There was also unbearable itchiness on my nose and around my eyes.

I later realized that the itchiness was not a good sign. It usually indicated the melanocytes were dying and the vitiligo was actively spreading. I couldn't help rubbing the itchy places and prematurely peeling off the dried skin. These actually accelerated the spreading, probably due to the Koebner phenomenon, which will be explained in chapter two. I stopped messing with the skin and instead used ice to relieve the itchiness thereafter.

Three years after my first visit to Dr. H, the condition on my face was getting out of hand; the white patches were expanding quickly. There were several big ones on my face and a small one on my neck. The white patches were so significant and embarrassing that I had to use some skin concealer whenever I went out.

I was extremely depressed when I pictured myself with a face full of those unsightly white patches. The psoralen was not working well and I didn't know what else to do.

SEARCHING FOR A SOLUTION

I felt helpless as the white patches were expanding every day. One morning, I looked into the mirror and said to myself, "I am not going to give up without a fight! I must do something! There must be something I can do! ".

As an engineer, I have many years of experiences in solving problems and finding solutions. To tackle a tough issue, the best way is to set up a project and put all your efforts in it.

So I started a project to look for a solution for my condition. When I searched for vitiligo treatments on the internet, the amount of information discovered was overwhelming. There were dozens of therapies and videos shared by fellow patients; there were hundreds of medical research papers; and of course there were a flood of advertisements for various drugs, therapies, and the so-called cures.

After reading many people's stories on their successful recovery, I realized that vitiligo could be healed and there were many things that I could try.

These stories lit up a fire of hope within me. I wholeheartedly thank those people who shared their stories and therapies, which were critical to my recovery.

THE EXCIMER LASER

I continued to read more medical research papers on the internet. I read about phototherapies using narrowband UVB (NBUVB) and the excimer lasers; I also read about the popular Protopic ointment and various other topical medications. I later found out that Protopic was one of the medicines prescribed to me by Dr. H years ago. That really surprised me. How come it didn't work for me?

I also read about how researchers combined Protopic and phototherapy to get better and faster repigmentation. Some patients and researchers even claimed that Protopic wouldn't work without sunlight or UVB exposure.

China has a lot of hospitals specializing in vitiligo treatment, but many have questionable credibility. During a trip to China, I visited a few hospitals in a city. I was not very satisfied with the first two. One doctor wanted to get me on the psoralen injections, which could cause pain and other side effects, for two months. The other wanted me to try a bunch of herb medicines that were quite inconvenient to prepare.

On the way back to the hotel, I saw a roadside advertisement for a vitiligo clinic. Such clinics are usually privately owned and many of them are known for ripping people off. However, I got curious and decided to check this one out. I figured I had nothing to lose if I wouldn't let my guard down, so I called a taxi.

To my surprise, this clinic was big, clean and professional looking, but awfully quiet with only a few patients in the huge lobby.

The girls at the front desk were very friendly. I signed in and was taken to a doctor's office a few minutes later.

I was assigned to Dr. F, who seemed to be a nice person and took his time explaining things. He checked my face and neck with a Wood's lamp. Upon my request, he even took a few pictures of the lesions using my own camera. Dr. F then ordered some tests: skin CT and blood work for trace elements.

I have had trace elements tested before and the results were normal; but have never heard about skin CT. In the lab on the second floor, a nurse rubbed some gel on my face and then pressed a sensor over the lesion area. A computer screen displayed the images captured. It felt similar to an ultrasonic scan procedure.

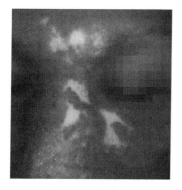

A picture taken under
the Wood's Lamp

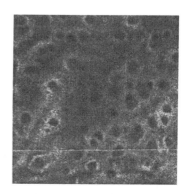

Skin CT Image

The test results were ready after 10 minutes. I was very impressed with their efficiency. In the previous two hospitals, I had to wait for hours to see a doctor.

Dr. F told me that the copper and zinc were marginally low in my blood, and the skin CT showed some half-moon shaped pigmentation, which he said was an indication of active vitiligo. However, there were still residual melanocytes or pigmentation within the white patches.

"This is good news," Dr. F said.

Then he moved on to introduce the treatment plan. He suggested combining some oral medicines with the 308-nm excimer laser phototherapy, which he claimed was the latest and the most effective technology in vitiligo treatment. As I had read about the excimer laser not too long ago, I knew he wasn't selling something bogus.

The cost of the treatment he proposed was quite high. The medication alone would cost about 200~300 dollars (yes, US dollars) a month. The fees for the phototherapy would be determined by the total area of the lesions, because each laser beam could only cover a small area, which was about 2cm x 2cm. For me, it would take eight beams to cover all the lesions, so the phototherapy charge would be at least 600 dollars a month. That was quite expensive, considering that many office workers in China made less than 800 dollars a month.

The treatment would usually last several months. It was impossible for me to stay there for an extended period of time. I told Dr. F politely that I needed to think this over. He seemed a little disappointed but was not upset.

"Well, it could be beneficial even if you had just one session of the laser treatment." Dr. F encouraged.

I was doubtful, but agreed to give it a shot. My philosophy was: if I tried new things, I would at least have some new experience and more chances in finding something that worked for me.

In the treatment room upstairs, a young nurse asked me to sit down as she adjusted the power level of the laser machine, which was about the size of a small washer and was made by a US company called PhotoMedex. The beam coming out of the treatment head was green. She asked me to close my eyes and then put the laser head near my face. I heard a few beeps as she was moving the laser from one spot to another and pushing the button. The laser beams felt warm and comfortable. In less than a minute, the session was painlessly done. I was told not to wash the treated area for the next two hours.

The next morning, I woke up and noticed the treated skin had turned pink and felt a little itchy. The pink tone also made the white patches less eye-catching. Two days later, I went there again to get another session on my way to the airport.

THE ELIDEL CREAM

The excimer laser seemed to have some effects, although it was really hard to tell after only two sessions. At my next stop, I visited another dermatologist in a state-owned hospital and got my third session of excimer laser treatment. I also asked the doctor to recommend some medications, but was told that the oral medications must be taken continuously for several months; otherwise it would be a waste of money.

I then asked for some Protopic ointment, and the doctor told me the hospital had only pimecrolimus (brand name Elidel), which I had not heard of or read about. According to the doctor, Elidel had been used in European trials and the results were quite positive.

The Elidel cream was not inexpensive and I didn't have a lot of local cash with me that day. I was going to say no, but changed my mind in seconds. My intuition told me that I should try this medicine.

This decision turned out to be a very important one.

I went back to the hotel and applied the Elidel cream on one of the white patches that night. Since I knew nothing about this cream, I decided to try it on a small lesion first.

I woke up the next morning and eagerly looked into the mirror. The lesion with the cream applied on appeared to be lighter and more noticeable than others!

"It made things worse!" Discouraged and disappointed, I threw the cream back into my suitcase.

I thought about this incident a few months later. The possible explanation was that the Elidel cream reduced the erythema (pinkish skin) caused by the laser treatment overnight and created a higher contrast between that lesion and the surrounding skin, making it more conspicuous. That was actually a positive thing, although in short-term it didn't look good.

Vitamin B12

I came back to US and started taking vitamin B12 and folic acid after reading about the vitamin B treatment study conducted by the Swedish researchers [1].

The trial conducted in Sweden used high dosage of vitamin B supplements: 10 mg (milligram) of folic acid and 2 mg of vitamin B12 daily. For the folic acid, 10 mg meant 25 of those 400 mcg (microgram) pills I could get from Walgreens. That seemed to be a lot, so I decided to cut it down.

I started taking 2000 mcg of vitamin B12 and 2000 mcg of folic acid daily. Occasionally, I would also take zinc (50 mg) and copper (2 mg) supplements. Later, I added calcium and fish oil to the regimen. A more detailed description of my treatment can be found in chapter five.

I made some fresh psoralen solution with 55% liquor and restarted the psoralen and sunlight combinational treatment. The psoralen treated areas would still give me a burning sensation and itchiness. Once the erythema disappeared, I saw only insignificant improvement. The healthy skin, if touched by the psoralen solution, would get much darker than the surrounding area.

The skin was still occasionally getting overexposed. With intense itchiness, the lesions were expanding again. The size of the lesions reached its peak at this point, and some lesions have crossed the center line of my face.

Back to the Elidel Cream

In despair, I dug out the Elidel cream from my suitcase and did some research on the internet. It turned out the cream was indeed used a lot in vitiligo treatment, although not as popular as Protopic, and was proved to be safe and effective for many patients. Knowing it wouldn't make things worse, I started using it twice a day regularly.

My scientific mind saw an opportunity to collect some firsthand medical experimental data here. Instead of using the cream on all the lesions, I decided to do some comparison experiments. For one patch, I applied nothing and used it to check how the vitamins worked alone; for another, I used the psoralen solution only; and I used the Elidel cream for the rest.

Based on the information from some medical research papers, I also sit in the morning or afternoon sun for at least 20 minutes every other day. I understood that combining Elidel or Protopic with UV phototherapy was not in accordance with the manufacturer's instructions, but I decided to take my chance since some medical researchers believed that the risks involved were limited. More information on this subject is available in chapter four.

The skin treated with the Elidel cream never bothered me after sunlight exposure. The skin might turn pink but it never itched or peeled off. The lesions did appear to be more conspicuous, because their borders had become darker and better defined. I looked at this as a positive thing: it meant the healthy skin around these lesions was fortifying its territories and closing in.

I also experimented with mixing Elidel and the psoralen on one patch. The skin treated with the mixture got a little thicker, from swelling perhaps, so I soon stopped this experiment.

After a few weeks, I did not see any negative impact from the Elidel cream, so I began applying it to all the lesions except one, which I reserved for comparison. From this point on, I completely stopped using the homemade psoralen solution because Elidel was working better for me.

CALLING PHOTOMEDEX

After coming back, I also started looking for nearby clinics that offered the 308-nm excimer laser phototherapy. I found a website established by PhotoMedex to help patients locate doctors and medical facilities that use their laser equipment.

I called the number on this website and was told there was a clinic that offered the excimer laser treatment in a plaza right next to where I live. Isn't that ironic? I went across the world to get laser treatments, and they are available half a mile away from my home.

Even though I believed the excimer laser was safe and would probably take care of the lesions on my face, I decided to experiment with other treatments first after considering the potential cost and some other factors. I reserved the excimer laser as my last line of defense.

The Diet Change

I have long noticed that the food I ate seemed to affect the vitiligo lesions. I also read stories of other vitiligo patients who got better simply by switching to healthier diets. Recently, CNN anchor Zain Verjee revealed how she got her severe psoriasis under control through rigid diet and meditation, after numerous failures with other treatments.

Diet therapy makes perfect sense because the food we eat closely interacts with our biological systems; therefore affecting our health. As a general principle, we should supply our bodies with the nutrients needed and eliminate the substances that are harmful. In addition, certain foods should not be mixed because they may react with each other and cause trouble.

My mom happens to be a person who has a lot of rules on what not to eat. For example, she won't eat beef or shrimp if she is dealing with pain or skin conditions; and she avoids radishes if she is taking medications. I had always shrugged off her rules in the past. However, I now decided to choose what I ate more carefully because the patches seemed to get itchy and larger after I ate certain foods.

I made some adjustments to my diet while using Elidel.

Shrimp was the first item I decided to eliminate from my diet. In Chinese medicine, shrimps and fish are considered detrimental for patients with skin conditions. Shrimps are also considered bottom feeders and forbidden food in many religions around the world. A recent report claimed that shrimps, especially the ones that were farmed and imported, were commonly contaminated with toxins and unapproved drugs.

I also decided to avoid very spicy food, which I had previously enjoyed from time to time. I remembered on two occasions the condition on my face got worse after I visited my hometown, where super spicy food was extremely popular and almost unavoidable. Although still using mild chili sauce occasionally, I stay clear of the extremely spicy items, such as jalapeño and hot red chili peppers.

Inspired by a conversation with Dr. Bob Lieberman, whom I met at a public speaking club, I started eating a clove of raw garlic every other day. Raw garlic can kill bad germs and is beneficial to the digestive system. This seemed to have improved my bowel movements. Be warned! Raw garlic can be very upsetting to the stomach. I would strongly suggest eating it with some food.

On top of these, I stopped eating or limited the consumption of things that were considered unhealthy, such as drinks with artificial color, canned food with preservatives, or anything else that I had doubt about.

I started drinking green tea more often because of its anti-oxidative properties, and stopped drinking water directly from the tap. I would drink boiled water, bottled natural spring water, and occasionally filtered water.

I also eat apples, watermelons, bananas, kiwis, pineapples, and oranges regularly. However, berries, especially blueberries, seem to give me a little trouble sometimes; so I usually go easy on them. Plus, berries are acid food.

After taking all these actions, my bowel movements got better and I have not experienced the itchiness on my face again. I believe diet management made a major contribution to my recovery by balancing my biological system and removing the issues that could have triggered vitiligo.

The Sun Exposure

In the first two years with vitiligo, I tried to stay away from direct sunlight whenever possible because I suspected the excessive sunlight exposure during commute and golfing might have triggered the initial depigmentation.

During my research, I read about the stories of several patients who recovered successfully. One thing in common was that they all had plenty of sunlight exposure, either on purpose or due to their jobs. Many studies have also proved that sunlight and NBUVB can accelerate the repigmentation process, especially when combined with topical or oral medicines. So it appears that the proper amount of sunlight exposure is beneficial to vitiligo recovery.

After knowing this, I stopped avoiding direct sunlight. I would make sure I got at least 20 minutes of direct sunlight exposure on the lesions every other day. Sometimes, I would even spend hours practicing or playing golf outdoors. However, I usually stay away from the mid-day sun because the UV is too strong around noon.

Sunlight is a free and viable UVB source. However, always carefully avoid overexposure, which may cause skin damage and even the spread of the lesions. If you are using the narrowband UVB light, dedicated sunlight exposure to the lesions is not a must, but getting in the natural spectrum of the sunlight once in a while is still beneficial.

The Turning Point

In the first two months of my new combinational therapy (vitamins, Elidel, sun exposure, and diet management), the improvement was insignificant, if any at all. Yet the situation was encouraging: the lesions stopped spreading.

About three months into the new therapy, I one day noticed that the white patches looked a little different. The borders got darker and clearer, and the patches appeared to be smaller! Some tiny brown spots were also showing up inside the bigger patches.

I was thrilled!

Then I started asking questions, "Why is it getting better? What could have contributed to the improvement? "

Once again my imagination went wild.

The first thing that came to my mind was a recent business trip. A few weeks before, I went to the city where I used to live for a meeting. I stayed in a hotel for one night, played a round of golf with a friend, and had a Greek pita and a Five Guys hamburger for dinner and lunch respectively. None of these seemed to be a possible triggering event.

Could it be the soap bar from the hotel? I used the soap to clean my face several times during the stay and at one point the bubbles got into my eyes and I still remembered the stinging pain. The traditional soap bars are alkaline. Didn't I read an article saying our bodies should stay alkaline to be healthy?

The soap probably wasn't the trigger. Nonetheless, I decided to put other facial cleansing products aside and started using the hotel-style plain soap bars to clean my face. I didn't know what kinds of chemicals were used in those fancy facial cleansing foams or gels; but I knew soap had a long history and a very good safety record.

Then, what else might have triggered the improvement?

I suddenly realized that I had been taking vitamins and using the Elidel cream for three months now, and the lesions that got noticeably better happened to be those on which I had applied the cream diligently. I also remembered that many researchers and patients on the internet mentioned "three months" a lot.

Could three months be the time it takes for the cream to do magic?

The patch that was not treated with the Elidel cream seemed to have improved less. I decided to put Elidel on it as well. Again, about three months later, this patch shrank significantly.

For the next few months, the first thing I did after getting up was to check the lesions with a magnifying mirror. And every day, I could see the lesions shrinking a little bit!

RECOVERING

After seven months of combinational therapy with Elidel, sun exposure, vitamin B and diet management, more than 80% of the affected areas on my face and neck had achieved repigmentation. I felt comfortable in public again without using any concealers.

Another good sign was that the skin itchiness had not happened again, a possible indication that the internal root cause for vitiligo was under control, most likely due to the diet management and the vitamin treatment.

Last but not the least, my digestive system got better. The frequency of abdominal pain and loose bowel movements significantly decreased. I believed that the raw garlic made its share of contribution.

THE PROTOPIC OINTMENT

My Elidel cream was running low and also approaching its expiration date. This small tube had lasted for about eight months now, and I was surprised. Even though the price of the cream was high, the average daily cost was quite insignificant.

I had planned to get both Protopic and Elidel to do some comparison. However, due to the availability issues, I eventually got only the Protopic 0.1% ointment and switched to it after Elidel ran out.

I didn't notice much of a difference after switching to the Protopic ointment other than the greasy looking skin. It was hard to compare the effectiveness from different periods anyway.

Personally, I have a slight preference for Elidel because it blends with skin better and also seems to have better coverage for the same amount. Protopic, on the other hand, makes the skin greasy, but it does stick to the skin better after sweating. It has been reported that Protopic was more effective in some trials.

The Narrowband UVB Light

Even though things were going in the right direction, I still decided to purchase a compact 311-nm narrowband UVB (NBUVB) light. I had a few reasons for this: first, there were days in which I wasn't able to get direct sunlight exposure because of the weather or my schedule; secondly, NBUVB is safer, purer and more effective than sunlight, which radiates a wider spectrum that includes the skin damaging and non-therapeutic wavelengths. Also, each phototherapy session with NBUVB takes only a few minutes, but would take 20-30 minutes with the sunlight; thirdly, I wanted to get some personal experience on how well NBUVB would work.

Most handheld NBUVB therapeutic kits at that time cost about 200~300 dollars each. Besides the NBUVB light, a kit usually includes a pair of UV protection eyewear and a digital timer. The key component of such a device is the NBUVB tube.

The lamp I got uses a Philips 9W NBUVB fluorescent tube (part number: PL-S 9W/01/2P), which was used in most of the handheld NBUVB devices in the market. The replacement tube itself costs about 45 dollars each. If someone sells it for much less, then there would be a good reason to suspect its authenticity because there are fake Philips NBUVB tubes out there.

I started using the NBUVB lamp every other day before I went to bed. Again, when trying something new, I usually test it at a small scale to get some experience. I first used the NBUVB to treat the lesions on my neck, along with the Protopic ointment.

I started with 30 seconds and progressively increased the exposure time to two and a half minutes after a few days, but still saw no erythema. That was a little odd. I then decided to remove the transparent plastic diffuser, which was placed over the NBUVB tube to even out the light. Without the diffuser, I started getting pink erythema on the lesions with two minutes of exposure time.

Previously, the lesions on my neck had recovered much slower than the ones on the face, but with the NBUVB I started seeing acceleration in repigmentation.

Not seeing any adverse effects for two weeks, I started treating all the lesions with the NBUVB light. Later, I changed the treatment frequency from every other day to three times a week.

WINNING THE BATTLE

After another four months, the stubborn lesions on my neck were completely gone! The lesions on my face achieved nearly complete repigmentation. There were still a couple of tiny faint spots left on my face. They were slowly gaining repigmentation and are barely noticeable now.

I have put together some pictures on the next page to demonstrate the healing process. I masked the eye areas with the mosaic effects, but no touch-up was done to the lesions. I also created a timeline chart showing how the lesions have changed over time, along with the treatments I used.

Looking back, the vitiligo experience was like a wakeup call to me. I learned a lot about healthy diets and healthy lifestyles, and I know I have to keep doing the right things to prevent the condition from happening again. I am happy and grateful that this special experience eventually ended on a good note and brought a positive spin to my life.

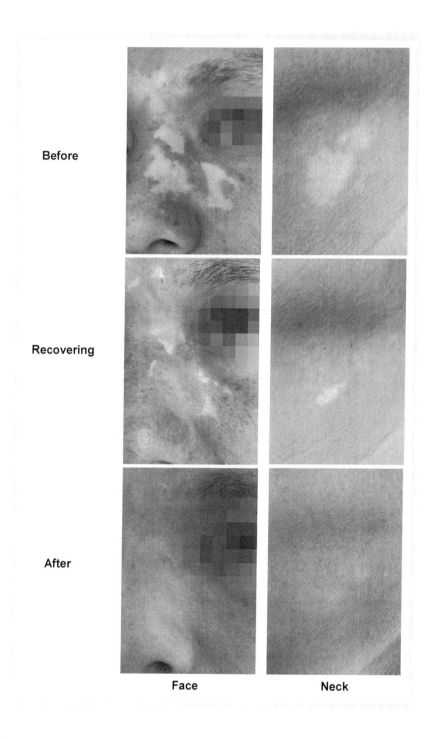

Before

Recovering

After

Face   Neck

20

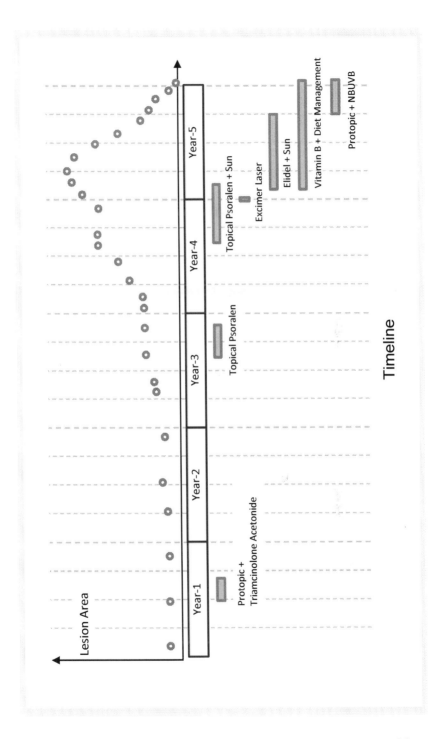

Timeline

21

2. Vitiligo Basics

If you are reading this book, chances are that you already know what vitiligo is. In a nutshell, vitiligo is a skin disorder in which the cells producing the skin pigmentation are disappearing, and white discoloration patches are formed on the skin. From a histological standpoint, a vitiligo lesion is characterized by the loss of pigment-producing cells in the absence of inflammation.

The percentage of the population affected by vitiligo varies in different areas and countries and is estimated to be 0.5~2%.

Males and females are equally affected and there is no apparent difference linked to skin types or races, although the lesions are more noticeable on people with darker skin.

The good news is that vitiligo is not contagious. However, contrary to the belief that these white patches are harmless to a patient's health, vitiligo usually is an indication that something is not right within one's biological system. In other words, vitiligo is rarely an isolated skin disorder; rather, it is often one of the symptoms of certain underlying health issues. This is perhaps the reason why vitiligo is considered difficult to treat: it won't go away, at least not for good, if it is only treated topically with the root causes of the problem ignored.

Even though the underlying issues might not be life-threatening, people should look at vitiligo as a warning sign, a wakeup call, and an opportunity to thoroughly evaluate their health conditions and make adjustments to their diets, lifestyles and living environments.

BASIC TERMINOLOGY

For a better understanding of the information discussed in the following chapters, some medical terms are briefly explained here. Readers can always acquire more information and knowledge from various online and offline sources.

Epidermis

The human skin is made of several layers, which are epidermis, dermis, and hypodermis from outside to inside.

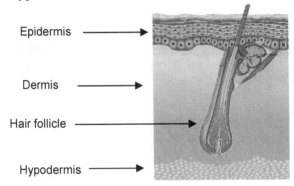

Epidermis

Dermis

Hair follicle

Hypodermis

Skin Structure

The epidermis is the external layer of the skin. It is an insensitive and nonvascular layer, which consists of 4~5 sub-layers. The top layer of the epidermis is called the stratum corneum, which is made of flat and dead skin cells. The bottom layer of the epidermis is where the pigment-producing cells are located and where the skin color is defined.

Dermis

The dermis is the inner layer of the skin that sits right under the epidermis. It is the sensitive and vascular layer where blood vessels, sweat glands, sebaceous glands, and nerves are located. The glands connect to the skin's surface through many tiny openings called pores. The hair follicles are also located in the dermis layer. It is believed that the hair follicles contain some reserved melanocytes, which can be activated to repair the vitiligo lesions.

Melanocyte

Melanocytes are the special cells that produce pigment for the skin and hair. The melanocytes for the skin reside at the bottom layer of the epidermis. They produce the protective pigment, which gives the skin different colors and protects the underlying tissues from UV damage.

There are about 1000~2000 melanocytes within one square millimeter of skin. Melanocytes comprise 5~10% of the cells in the basal layer of the epidermis.

Melanin

Melanin is produced by melanocytes and is the pigment that defines the color of the skin. Melanin can also be found in hairs and eyes. UV irradiation can stimulate melanogenesis, which is the process of producing melanin. Melanin absorbs and blocks UV rays to protect the tissues under the skin from DNA damage.

In vitiligo, the depigmentation is caused by the absence or reduction of melanocytes. As a comparison, in some other skin disorders, such as albinism, the melanocytes are still in place; it is the melanin production that is compromised.

Autoimmunity

The human body has a sophisticated immune system to protect itself from diseases and the invasion of external bacteria and viruses.

Sometimes things can go wrong, and the immune system would mistakenly identify the body's own cells and tissues as enemies and launch attacks to destroy them. Such self-attacking activities are called autoimmunity. A disease caused by the autoimmune responses is called an autoimmune disease.

An autoimmune disease may affect any tissue or organ, including skin, joints, muscles, glands, digestive tract, and blood vessels. Examples of autoimmune diseases include:

- Addison's disease
- Hashimoto's thyroiditis
- Pernicious anemia
- Reactive arthritis
- Rheumatoid arthritis
- Vitiligo
- Psoriasis
- Systemic lupus erythematosus
- Diabetes (type 1)

To treat autoimmune disorders, immunosuppressants are commonly prescribed to reduce the activities of the immune system. Corticosteroids and calcineurin inhibitors are examples of immunosuppressants.

T Cells

T cells, also called T lymphocytes, are the key components of the human immune system. T cells are in fact a type of white blood cell that matures in the thymus, for which the T stands.

T cells are divided into helper T cells, which regulate the immune responses, and killer T cells, which attack those cells that carry certain foreign or abnormal molecules on their surfaces. Killer T cells are equipped with potent chemicals that are used to attack and destroy the targeted objects.

T cells are associated with allergic reactions, organ transplant rejection, and autoimmune diseases. In one of the theories for vitiligo, T cells are believed to have mistakenly targeted and killed the pigment-producing melanocytes.

Koebner Phenomenon / Isomorphic Response

The Koebner phenomenon, also known as the isomorphic response, refers to the development of new lesions of an existing skin disease on a traumatized but previously healthy skin area.

The Koebner phenomenon was first described by Heinrich Koebner, a German dermatologist, in 1872. Dr. Koebner noticed that new lesions would form on previously healthy skin after skin trauma (cuts, punctures, friction, bug bites, etc.) for some psoriasis patients. The immune response at the newly injured skin was believed to have caused the new lesions.

In a case reported recently, a psoriasis patient experienced an outbreak of new lesions after getting acupuncture for his back pain. Previously, he had lesions on his arms and legs only. The new lesions appeared on his lower back, the exact location where the acupuncture was performed. In another case, a patient developed new psoriasis lesions two weeks after getting tattoos on his arms.

The Koebner phenomenon may also happen with many other skin disorders, including vitiligo and lichen planus. Usually, the new lesions would occur a couple of weeks after the skin injury.

During the active stage of vitiligo, patients should be extremely careful about the Koebner phenomenon and try to avoid skin trauma such as:

- Cuts
- Sunburns
- Forceful scratching or rubbing
- Tattoos
- Acupuncture
- Bug or animal bites

WHAT HAPPENS IN VITILIGO

There have been different opinions on what really happens within the vitiligo lesions. Does vitiligo happen because the melanocytes stop producing melanin or because the melanocytes are gone? For certain skin disorders involving discoloration, the melanocytes are still in place but unable to produce any melanin. Is this the case with vitiligo? Knowing what is actually going on is important to finding the right treatments.

Several studies have so far confirmed that vitiligo lesions are characterized by the disappearance of melanocytes. In 1993, a research group in Netherlands investigated into this subject using immunohistochemistry and concluded that the depigmentation in vitiligo was indeed caused by the loss of melanocytes.

However, this does not mean that all the melanocytes are gone. In 2000, a group in UK confirmed the existence of residual melanocytes in vitiligo lesions, including those that have been stable for as long as 25 years [2]. They were able to restore the function of the residual melanocytes by removing hydrogen peroxide (H_2O_2), which causes oxidative stress, from the skin.

This is an encouraging fact for vitiligo patients. It means vitiligo depigmentation is reversible.

WHAT CAUSES VITILIGO

Although many hypotheses or theories have been proposed, the exact causes of vitiligo are not clearly known or understood by the medical community as of today. The pathogenesis of vitiligo can be complicated and the exact root causes or triggers may not be the same for all patients.

The commonly discussed theories or hypotheses on what causes vitiligo include autoimmune disorder, oxidative overstress, and genetic defects, etc.

Autoimmune Disorder

There is increasing evidence that certain autoimmune mechanism is involved in vitiligo. It was reported that activated T cells and melanocyte antigens were frequently detected around the active vitiligo lesions.

It has been reported that autoimmune disorders, especially those related to the thyroid, are more prevalent in vitiligo patients than in the general population, indicating a possible connection between the two. Autoimmune thyroid diseases, such as Hashimoto thyroiditis, have been reported as the most frequent autoimmune disorders associated with vitiligo.

In this theory, the T cells are activated mistakenly to attack the melanocytes and induce their self-destruction, which in turn causes the depigmentation patches on the skin. Based on this theory, immunosuppressants are used to curb the overly active immune response and to stop the T cells from attacking the melanocytes.

However, it is not unreasonable to postulate that autoimmunity is perhaps just a step at the end of a complex chain reaction. It might actually be the consequence of some other activities, rather than the root cause of the whole situation.

Oxidative Stress

The metabolic processes in our bodies consume oxygen to generate energy. At the same time, they produce byproducts: free radicals, which are reactive molecules with unpaired electrons. The most concerning radicals are called Reactive Oxygen Species (ROS), which are derived from oxygen molecules.

With their high reactivity, ROS can be used to attack the harmful invaders in our bodies. On the other hand, they can also interact with and cause damage to our own molecules and cells.

Our bodies have defense mechanisms that can produce antioxidants to neutralize the excessive ROS and repair the damage they incur. However, if there are not enough antioxidants to maintain the balance, excessive ROS will wonder around and cause harmful effects. Such a state is called oxidative stress.

Oxidative stress is blamed for many diseases, including Parkinson's disease, autism, and chronic fatigue syndrome. It could also affect melanocytes and interfere with the melanogenesis process,

28

and consequently cause vitiligo. Significant depletion of antioxidants has been reported in the epidermis of active vitiligo patients.

We can change our diets, lifestyles, and living environments to reduce the level of oxidative stress. Foods, such as artichokes, beans, and apples, are rich in antioxidants. Vitamin E is a lipid-soluble antioxidant and can protect membranes from oxidative damage. Vitamin C can also reduce radicals that come from a variety of sources.

Catalase is an antioxidant enzyme that also can reduce oxidative stress. It can degrade hydrogen peroxide, which is a type of ROS, to water and oxygen. Studies have showed that catalase could be low and inactive in patients with an elevated epidermis hydrogen peroxide level.

Based on this theory, topical pseudocatalases, which can lower the levels of hydrogen peroxide and help reduce oxidative stress, have been proposed for vitiligo treatment with or without UVB. A German group conducted a pilot study and achieved success on treating vitiligo patients with topical application of pseudocatalase and calcium, along with short-term UVB light exposure [3].

Genetic Factor

Another hypothesis is that genetic factors might also have played an important role in the development of vitiligo. Researchers studied the pattern of familial aggregation of vitiligo and concluded the extent of genetic factor involvement is statistically significant.

The onset of vitiligo seems to require environmental triggers, such as foods, drinks, pollution, or stress, even for people who are genetically susceptible.

Genetic factors, when combined with environmental triggers, may contribute to the loss of immune tolerance and the attack to the melanocytes by the immune system.

Other Influences

Many doctors claim that vitiligo is a noncontagious cosmetic issue that does not affect the patients' general health. Opinions like this can be misleading.

Vitiligo is the visible indication, or a symptom, of certain underlying health issues. Almost every vitiligo patient has some other health concerns and might be in the so-called sub-health state. However, such underlying issues may not be severe, and therefore do not usually get the attention they deserve. The patients often consider themselves healthy other than having some skin imperfections. Or such issues may not appear to be relevant to a skin disorder, so people usually fail to connect the dots between them.

It has come to my attention that some vitiligo patients, including myself, also suffer from digestive issues. One female patient reported that her vitiligo recovered after the digestive issues were taken care of. Obviously, stories like this strengthened my speculation that my vitiligo might have been triggered by the digestive tract disorders, which started about one year before the onset of my vitiligo. It was unfortunate that none of the doctors I had visited was able to diagnose the issue, or was interested in doing so.

Medical studies have discovered that digestive tract issues could cause the loss of, or the inability to absorb, certain critical nutrients, therefore can trigger mysterious health problems.

Could vitiligo be one of these mysterious problems?

The Leaky Gut

Another interesting topic related to the digestive tract is the Leaky Gut Syndrome. Healthy intestines can screen out the harmful substances and only absorb properly digested nutrients. For some people, the walls of the intestines are damaged and become more permeable, allowing undigested food, bacteria, or waste to sneak into the bloodstream without proper screening.

Consequently, the immune system responds to the invasion of these unexpected objects and launches attacks to get rid of them, causing inflammation, allergy, or even autoimmune disorders.

Also, for people with leaky guts, the intestine lining is damaged and not capable of producing certain enzymes needed to break down the food for proper digestion. They become sensitive or allergic to certain foods that healthy people would benefit from.

The symptoms of leaky gut syndrome vary. Typical ones include multiple food sensitivities, nutritional deficiency, chronic diarrhea, headaches, fatigue, etc.

Probiotics can help the good bacteria in the intestines grow back and heal the gut lining. Fish oil and zinc supplements can help strengthen the intestine walls.

According to the experiences of many people, leaky gut can also be treated through diet management.

The Air Conditioner Analogy

One hot summer afternoon, the AC in my house decided to take a break. Our home felt like a huge sauna.

The outcome of a broken AC system is the same: high room temperature. Yet there are hundreds of possible causes for the same symptom. It can be caused by an inexpensive fuse or a costly motor.

This time the problem was quite strange: if I shut down the AC for a couple hours and restarted it, it would put out cool air for about 10 minutes and then failed again. I knew from my experience that these intermittent issues were very difficult to troubleshoot. The problem would often come back right after the service technician left. I was enticed by this strange issue and decided to check it out myself before calling a service company.

Both the thermostat and the indoor unit (air handler) appeared to be working properly, but the fan in the outdoor unit (compressor) was not running. The fan motor had failed before and was replaced once, so the first thought came to my mind was that the motor might have failed again. A replacement motor would cost at least 300 dollars.

Instead of blaming the motor right away, I did more inspection and discovered that the controller was not always sending out the signal to turn on the compressor. Here came my second thought: the controller could be broken. That also meant expensive replacement parts.

Further investigation revealed that the controller didn't send out the signal because something stopped it from doing so: the safety switch was triggered because the pipe that drained the condensate from the indoor unit was blocked and caused the condensate to overflow!

It turned out the drain pipe was clogged at the other end outside the house. I cut the end off the pipe, cleaned it up and put it back together. Viola! We got cool air again without having to replace any parts!

Why would the AC work for about 10 minutes after being shut down for a while? Because with the AC turned off, the condensate would evaporate and lower the water level. This allowed the safety switch to reset. After 10 minutes of operation, the condensate level rose again and retriggered the safety switch. I could bypass the safety switch, just like suppressing the immune system with medicines, to get the cool air back, but that would be causing a wet floor later.

Without careful investigation, I could have spent several hundred dollars to replace the motor and the controller, and still ended up with the problem unsolved.

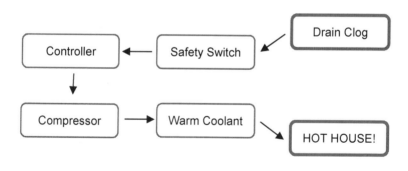

AC Failure Chain Reaction

What is the point of this story? The failure of a complex system could be triggered by a tiny issue hidden behind a complex chain reaction. Each link in the chain might have appeared to be the culprit at first glance; but only by careful analysis can one pinpoint the root cause of the failure.

The onset of vitiligo could be of the same nature. The similar looking white patches might have been triggered by some seemingly irrelevant health issues, which can be specific to each patient. The autoimmunity or the oxidative stress could just be a step near the end of the chain reaction, and therefore might not be the actual root cause of the condition. If this is the case, topical treatments targeting the vitiligo lesions directly might not be the ultimate solution.

Each vitiligo patient can benefit from a thorough review of his health conditions. Some of the chronic issues might be related to the onset of his vitiligo.

DIFFERENT TYPES OF VITILIGO

Vitiligo can be categorized into different types. Being familiar with the types of vitiligo can help patients narrow down the possible causes and choose the proper treatments.

Overall, vitiligo can be classified as *segmental* and *non-segmental* types. The lesion distribution of segmental vitiligo is usually restrained to one side of the body. Non-segmental vitiligo lesions happen on both sides of the body. Some patients can have both segmental and non-segmental vitiligo features and are considered to have a mixed type.

Vitiligo can also be classified by the area involved: localized, generalized, and universal. However, such classifications do not seem to reflect the essential difference among different types.

Segmental Vitiligo

The lesions of segmental vitiligo are usually restricted to a segment on one side of the body and rarely cross the center line. The distribution of the lesions is usually associated with one or more dermatomes. A dermatome is an area of skin that is under the control of a particular spinal nerve. More than 50% of the segmental vitiligo patients have lesions on their face. Some patients have lesions on both their face and neck.

Segmental vitiligo usually starts at an early age, and tends to stabilize after a period of quick development. Segmental vitiligo is not typically considered to have association with autoimmune disorders, although a small percentage of patients may have thyroid disease, diabetes, or atopic dermatitis. About half of the patients also have white hairs within the lesions, often on their heads or eyebrows.

Non-segmental Vitiligo

Non-segmental vitiligo, which is also known as vitiligo vulgaris, has lesions distributed on both sides of the body, often symmetrically. Non-segmental vitiligo often has connections with autoimmune diseases such as thyroid disorders, diabetes mellitus, and Addison's disease. Non-segmental vitiligo can happen at any age with an unpredictable course of development, which may continue throughout a patient's lifetime.

Non-segmental vitiligo and segmental vitiligo may coexist on the same patient and such is referred to as the mixed type. Non-segmental vitiligo or the mixed type is more commonly seen among vitiligo patients. According to some medical experts, segmental vitiligo is relatively easier to treat than the non-segmental type.

DIFFERENT STAGES OF VITILIGO

Vitiligo can be at different stages of its development: the active stage where it is still progressing; or the stable stage where it is under control.

Knowing the difference is of great importance in choosing the right treatments and caring strategies. Patients at the active stage may

34

need special medications to help control the quick spread of the lesions. They must also watch for the Koebner phenomenon. Some treatments are only suitable for patients at the stable stage, and could worsen the condition or be less effective if used during the active stage.

For example, the success rate of suction blister grafting surgery has close relation to the duration of stability. A patient that had been stable for less than one year often exhibited poor repigmentation, whereas nearly 78% of those who had been stable for more than two years had very successful repigmentation.

Active Stage

During the active stage, melanocytes are dying, existing vitiligo lesions are getting bigger, and new lesions are developing. Patients may feel remarkable itchiness and burning on or around the skin affected. Visually, the borders of the lesions are obscure.

During the active stage, skin trauma may trigger new vitiligo lesions due to the Koebner phenomenon. Patients should resist the temptation to forcefully scratch the itchy skin around the lesions, and carefully avoid sunburns, cuts and other skin injuries.

The treatment strategy for active vitiligo is usually different from that used in the stable stage. During the active stage, doctors may use systemic immunomodulators or immunosuppressants to control the progression. Topical photosensitizers and UV treatments should be used with caution. Extended sunlight exposure and high doses of NBUVB should be avoided because severe erythema might trigger new lesions. However, excimer laser is considered safe to use in the active stage because it can inhibit T cell activities.

Stable Stage

The stable stage refers to a period when the underlying mechanism causing vitiligo is under control, either temporarily or permanently. The stabilization can result from the removal or reduction of the factors that triggered the vitiligo onset in the first place.

At present, the medical community has no consensus on the criteria for the stable stage. In the past, clinical characteristics were relied upon; now biochemical and ultra-structural features are also considered as the technologies improve. The most accepted criteria are as follows:

- The existing lesions are not getting bigger
- There are no new lesions
- The borders of the existing lesions are well-defined
- The patient experiences no Koebner phenomenon

Recovering Stage

During the recovering stage, the issues that triggered vitiligo onset have been eliminated and conditions that facilitate melanocyte revival and growth are present. As a result, the melanocytes along the borders migrate towards the centers of the lesions, and the residual melanocytes grow back from inside. This is evidenced by the shrinking vitiligo lesions and the small repigmentation islands inside them.

UVB exposure usually has a positive role in the recovering stage. A proper level of sunlight or artificial UVB exposure is known to assist and accelerate the recovering process.

BLOOD TEST FOR VITAMINS AND TRACE ELEMENTS

According to the findings of some medical studies, the thyroid function, blood cell counts, vitamin levels, and trace element levels in the blood are normal for most vitiligo patients. Therefore, the results of such tests are not always meaningful or definitive in vitiligo diagnosis [4].

RESPONSE TO TREATMENT

A universal cure for vitiligo is yet to be found. The effectiveness of the treatments currently available depends on the specific conditions of each patient. A treatment may work very well for some patients but not at all for others. This is probably because the exact causes or triggers for vitiligo can be different for a specific group of patients.

How a vitiligo lesion responds to a particular treatment is also highly dependent on its location. As reported by many studies, lesions on the face and neck are the most responsive to treatments and usually have a higher rate of complete repigmentation. This is a good thing because lesions on the face and neck probably have the most severe impact on an individual's social live.

It is believed that the hair follicles on the face and neck have reserved melanocytes, which can be revived to grow and migrate. Also, the face and the neck are frequently exposed to sunlight, which helps the repigmentation. Conversely, the lesions on the bony areas or the extremities, such as the hands and feet, are less responsive to current treatments.

3. Medications for Vitiligo

INTRODUCTION

A lot of oral and topical medicines, as well as dietary supplements are used in vitiligo treatment today. This chapter will give the readers an overview of the commonly used items so they can make better decisions and communicate with their doctors more effectively.

In general, the medicines and supplements used in vitiligo treatment fall under the following categories:

- Immunomodulators
- Calcineurin inhibitors
- Corticosteroids
- Photosensitizers
- Vitamins
- Others

IMMUNOMODULATORS

Immunomodulators are usually used to control the quick progression of vitiligo during the active stage. The use of immunomodulators must be under the supervision of a qualified physician. People who have liver issues should inform their doctors of the conditions and be cautious in using the medicines in this category.

Pidotimod

Pidotimod is a synthesized immunomodulator. In vitiligo treatment, pidotimod is usually used to control the progression of vitiligo.

Many companies offer pidotimod in the form of granules or oral solution. *Polimod* is a brand name pidotimod produced by an Italian company. It is considered by many medical practitioners as a safe and high quality pidotimod option.

Pidotimod is available to patients in Italy, China, Mexico, Costa Rica, South Korea, and Greece, etc. Currently, it appears that pidotimod is available for medical research only in US.

Transfer Factor

Transfer factors are small molecules that can transfer the immunity against certain diseases from one system to another. As immunomodulators, they can help modulate and balance the immune system.

In 1949, American immunologist Dr. H. Sherwood Lawrence of New York University discovered that the immune response carried by lymphocytes extract could be transferred from one body to another to enhance the latter's immune system.

In 1998, an American company introduced to the market a line of transfer factor products that were produced from cow colostrum, which is the milk secreted by a cow in the first few days after giving birth. Its scientists later discovered that eggs also contained transfer factors and the combination of the two increased the effectiveness dramatically.

Transfer factors can be used to treat certain skin conditions, including psoriasis, atopic dermatitis, and many others. Some doctors have used it to treat vitiligo, especially to control the progression of active vitiligo.

Transfer factor capsules are available in drugstores as over-the-counter dietary supplements.

Calcineurin Inhibitors

Calcineurin inhibitors, which are a type of immunosuppressant, can suppress the body's immune activities and are commonly used in organ transplantation to prevent rejection.

The two most popular topical calcineurin inhibitors for vitiligo treatment are Protopic and Elidel, whose active ingredients are tacrolimus and pimecrolimus respectively. Throughout the rest of this book, Protopic and tacrolimus are considered interchangeable, so are Elidel and pimecrolimus. Most of medical papers use the generic names, but I tend to use the brand names when talking about specific applications.

Calcineurin is a protein phosphatase that activates the T cells, which are considered to have major contribution to the death of melanocytes in vitiligo lesions. As the name implies, calcineurin inhibitors can reduce the activation of T cells by blocking calcineurin, therefore preventing the attacks on the melanocytes.

Calcineurin inhibitors can boost the migration of melanocytes and stimulate melanogenesis. Furthermore, they are also known to inhibit the production of reactive oxygen species and thus prevent the destruction of melanocytes by oxidative stress, which was previously discussed in chapter two.

According to a medical research paper [4], some patients who did not respond to corticosteroids achieved complete repigmentation after using topical tacrolimus ointment and getting mild exposure to natural sunlight for 2~4 months. Calcineurin inhibitors also make the skin more sensitive to light. However, they won't cause skin thinning as the corticosteroids do.

Protopic (tacrolimus)

Protopic is a brand name calcineurin inhibitor ointment produced by Japanese company Astellas Toyama. Its active ingredient is tacrolimus, which is a type of immunosuppressant. Protopic is a prescription medicine that was originally used for treating eczema.

Now it is a famous and widely used medicine in vitiligo treatment.

Protopic is available in two different strengths: 0.1% and 0.03%. According to the manufacturer, adults may use either Protopic ointment 0.1% or 0.03%; but children between 2 and 15 years of age should only use Protopic ointment 0.03%. Protopic should not be used on children younger than 2 years of age.

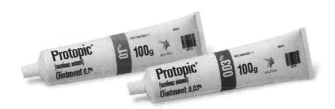

Protopic Ointment

Patients can choose from 10g, 30g, 60g, and 100g packages. It is better to get smaller packages because it is not advisable to keep an opened tube for an extended period of time.

Elidel (pimecrolimus)

Elidel is another brand name calcineurin inhibitor commonly used for eczema and vitiligo treatment. Elidel is manufactured by Novartis in Germany. Its active ingredient is pimecrolimus.

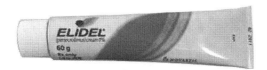

Elidel Cream

Although having similar functions as Protopic, Elidel comes in the form of cream, which bonds with skin better and can be absorbed faster. The Protopic ointment, on the other hand, has a slight disadvantage with absorption, but it stays on the skin longer because it won't be washed off easily by the sweat or water.

Elidel is available in 1% strength only, and comes in 15g, 30g, 60g, and 100g packages. The instruction suggests discarding the cream after it has been opened for more than 12 months. For people who use only a small amount daily, it is a good idea to get the smaller packages.

Comparison

In treating atopic dermatitis, both medications are equally effective with patients of mild condition; but patients with moderate-to-severe conditions had significantly greater improvement with tacrolimus 0.1% than pimecrolimus 1% according to a randomized study involving 1065 patients [5].

One study [6] reported that a significant reduction of oxidative stress and an increase of antioxidant capacity in the serum were observed in vitiligo patients treated with topical tacrolimus. Pimecrolimus, however, did not induce such changes.

Several studies have reported that tacrolimus was more efficacious than pimecrolimus in clinical trials; while some others did not observe much difference.

Compared to tacrolimus, pimecrolimus has higher lipophilicity, which means it dissolves easier in fats and lipids and therefore can be absorbed better.

Safety

In general, both tacrolimus and pimecrolimus are safe and well tolerated by patients. Both have very low incidence of side effects. The common short-term side effects include temporary erythema and burning sensation at the application sites. Unlike the irreversible skin atrophy caused by the topical corticosteroids, the side effects of tacrolimus and pimecrolimus usually only happen in the first few days of usage. More safety information, including the FDA advisory and black box warning, will be discussed in chapter four.

The medication guides for Protopic and Elidel both suggest that they should be used for short periods. If needed, treatment may be repeated with breaks in between.

The medication guides further suggest that during the course of treatment, patients should minimize sunlight exposure and avoid ultraviolet light therapy. It is not known whether these two medicines interfere with the skin's response to ultraviolet damage.

However, many doctors and researchers have combined Protopic or Elidel with phototherapy (sunlight, NBUVB, or excimer laser, etc.) and discovered that the combinational therapy was much more effective than either one alone. More details will be provided in chapter four.

CORTICOSTEROIDS

Corticosteroids are a class of drugs that are commonly used to decrease inflammation and suppress immune system activities. They are also a type of immunosuppressant.

Corticosteroids have long been used to treat allergic reactions such as asthma and atopic dermatitis (eczema). Since corticosteroids are similar to cortisol, the hormone naturally produced by the adrenal gland, they are also used to treat diseases in which a person's adrenal gland does not produce enough hormones.

Corticosteroids can be given topically or systemically (oral, IV, or muscle injection). Systemic corticosteroid treatment has also been used by doctors to control the rapid progression of active vitiligo.

Topical corticosteroids used to be the main medicines for vitiligo before tacrolimus and pimecrolimus were available, and are effective for some patients.

Topical corticosteroids come with different potencies. The

highly potent ones should not be used on the face. The topical corticosteroids commonly used for vitiligo are listed below:

- Clobetasol Propionate 0.05%
- Betamethasone Dipropionate 0.05%
- Halometasone
- Mometasone Furoate 0.1%
- Clotrimazole and Betamethasone Dipropionate
- Triamcinolone Acetonide 0.1%
- Hydrocortisone Butyrate 0.1%
- Methylprednisolone

Safety

The risk of severe side effects is high with corticosteroids. Long-term use of topical corticosteroids may cause irreversible skin thinning (atrophy). Usually, topical corticosteroids should not be used continuously for more than two or three months, depending on the potency.

PHOTOSENSITIZERS

Photosensitizers are used to increase the skin's sensitivity to UV rays, promote melanocyte's growth, and stimulate the melanogenesis process. There are several types of photosensitizers for vitiligo treatment.

Psoralen (Methoxsalen)

Psoralen can be taken orally or applied topically to enhance the skin's photosensitivity. Psoralen is commonly combined with UVA phototherapy to achieve repigmentation in a traditional treatment known as PUVA (Psoralen + UVA), which was once the golden-standard in vitiligo treatment.

The side effects of oral psoralen are quite significant. The whole body of the patient who takes oral psoralen will become photosensitive. After the treatment, he must keep his whole body, especially his eyes, from direct sunlight to avoid overexposure. Consequently, PUVA with oral psoralen is no longer considered a preferred treatment nowadays.

PUVA with topical psoralen only affects the skin treated, and won't cause any harm to other parts of the body. This option is safer and has fewer side effects.

A commonly used drug in the psoralen group is methoxsalen, which is also known as 8-Methoxypsoralen, 8-MOP or Oxsoralen.

Methoxsalen shall be used under the close supervision of a qualified physician. It is not recommended for children younger than 12 years of age.

Homemade Topical Psoralen Solution

Babchi (psoralea corylifolia) seeds contain psoralen and have photosensitization effects. They are similar to black peppers in size and color.

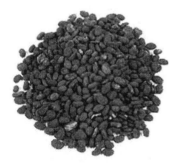

Bachi Seeds

Homemade topical psoralen solution can be produced by soaking one part of babchi seeds in two parts of 75% alcohol or high density liquor for one or two weeks. This solution is a viable option for people who have limited access to prescription medications or other more costly treatments.

Khellin

Khellin is a constituent extracted from khella, which is a flowering plant also known as ammi visnaga. Tea prepared from the fruits of khella has been traditionally used to treat kidney stones in Egypt.

Essentially, khellin is a furanochromone and chemically similar to psoralen. It has been used as a photosensitizer to treat vitiligo with some success. It makes the skin sensitive to UV rays and can stimulate melanocyte activities.

Khellin is supposed to be used along with UV irradiation and has comparable efficacy to psoralen. However, unlike psoralen, khellin does not induce skin phototoxic erythema according to a medical study conducted by an Austrian group [7], and is considered safer than psoralen.

Khellin can be given topically, orally, or through IV. However, it was reported that oral or IV khellin could cause liver transaminase elevation and nausea [7][8].

VITAMINS

Vitamins, especially vitamin B supplements, have been used to treat vitiligo with encouraging results. Vitamin B12 and vitamin B9 (folate or folic acid) are among the most important ones.

Vitamin B12

Vitamin B12, also called cobalamin, is required for proper red blood cell formation, neurological function, and DNA synthesis. It is vital for maintaining healthy nerve cells. Vitamin B12 also works together with folate to produce SAMe, a compound involved in immune function. The combination of vitamin B12 and folate has been used to treat vitiligo by many patients with positive outcomes.

Vitamin B12 deficiency can cause fatigue, diarrhea, anemia, nerve damages, etc. For men, it can also cause low sperm count and poor sperm mobility.

Vitamin B12 naturally exists in a wide variety of animal foods. Major sources of vitamin B12 include:

- Clams
- Beef livers
- Fish
- Eggs
- Dairy products

Vitamin B12 can also be acquired through dietary supplements and is usually available in three forms:

- Cyanocobalamin
- Hydroxocobalamin
- Methylcobalamin

Supplement Facts

Serving Size 1 Tablet

	Amount Per Serving	% Daily Value
Vitamin B12 (as cyanocobalamin)	1000 mcg	16,670%

Vitamin B12: Cyanocobalamin

Cyanocobalamin is the least expensive and the most used form in various vitamin B12 and multivitamin supplements. It has to be converted to the active forms, such as methylcobalamin, inside our bodies to be useful. Many opinions consider methylcobalamin a better and preferred form of vitamin B12 supplement.

Supplement Facts

Serving Size 1 Tablet

	Amount Per Serving	% Daily Value
Vitamin B12 (as methylcobalamin)	1000 mcg	16,667%

Vitamin B12: Methylcobalanmin

Since vitamin B12 does not exist in the plant foods, strict vegetarians should take vitamin B12 supplements to avoid deficiency.

Folate, Folic Acid

Although often used interchangeably, folate and folic acid are chemically different forms of vitamin B9.

Folate is the form of vitamin B9 that is naturally present in many foods. Unlike vitamin B12, folate can be found in both plant and animal foods, including:

- Beef livers, chicken livers
- Spinach, lettuce, broccoli
- Asparagus, Brussels sprouts
- Avocados, tomatoes, oranges, bananas

Folic acid, on the other hand, often refers to a synthetic form of vitamin B9 that is commonly seen in dietary supplements and fortified foods. Folate can be directly metabolized in the small intestines, whereas folic acid will have to first go through its initial conversion in the liver.

Folate deficiency usually coexists with some other nutrient deficiencies. In addition to anemia, it can also cause pigmentation changes in skin, hair, and fingernails.

Adequate folate is essential to our health. Women with insufficient folate intakes are at increased risk of giving birth to infants with neural tube defects. For this reason, folate or folic acid is often taken by women who plan to have children to prevent birth defects.

According to publications from the National Institutes of Health, folate from natural foods may lower the risks of several forms of cancers.

Getting folate through natural foods is the best and the safest choice. Folate is also available as dietary supplements; it is usually labeled as 5-methyltetrahydrofolate or 5-MTHF and is a better form than folic acid. The following picture shows the fact sheet of a folate supplement.

Supplement Facts

Serving Size 1 Capsule   Servings Per Container 60

	Amount Per Serving	% DV
Folate (as Quatrefolic® (6S)-5-methyltetrahydrofolic acid glucosamine salt)	400 mcg	100%

Folate Capsule

Folic acid is commonly used in B-complex vitamins or multi-vitamins. The following chart shows that folic acid, not folate, is used in this B-100 vitamin supplement.

Supplement Facts

Serving Size 1 Capsule

Amount Per Serving		%Daily Value
Thiamin (Vitamin B-1) (as Thiamin Mononitrate)	100 mg	6,667%
Riboflavin (Vitamin B-2)	100 mg	5,882%
Niacin (as Niacinamide)	100 mg	500%
Vitamin B-6 (as Pyridoxine Hydrochloride)	100 mg	5,000%
Folic Acid	400 mcg	100%
Vitamin B-12 (as Cyanocobalamin)	100 mcg	1,667%
Biotin	100 mcg	33%
Pantothenic Acid (as d-Calcium Pantothenate)	100 mg	1,000%

B-complex Capsule

Vitamin B12 usually goes hand in hand with folate or folic acid in vitiligo treatment. They should be taken together to be safe and effective. Taking a high dose of folate or folic acid alone can prevent anemia and this may hide the symptoms of a potential vitamin B12 deficiency and allow permanent nerve damage to develop without warning. A mild B12 deficiency, even though not enough to cause anemia, may still impair brain functions.

A long-term and high level intake of folic acid has raised some concerns because unmetabolized folic acid can enter the bloodstream and might cause issues. Modest amounts of folic acid taken before a cancer develops might decrease cancer risks, but high doses of folic acid taken after the cancer (especially colorectal cancer) begins might speed up its progression. For this reason, a high dosage (1000 mcg or greater) of folic acid supplement should be taken with caution.

Although many of the medical papers concerning vitiligo treatment used the term folic acid, folate is a better option when taken at high dosage for an extended period of time.

Oral vitamin B12 and folic acid, in combination with sunlight exposure, have been reported to deliver positive results in vitiligo treatment.

Vitamin C

The role of vitamin C in vitiligo treatment is controversial. Supposedly, vitamin C functions as an antioxidant and can help reduce oxidative stress. There are doctors who believe vitamin C consumption is beneficial to the repigmentation process; and they encourage patients to take vitamin C supplements and eat vitamin rich foods.

Then there are some other doctors who believe vitamin C is harmful to vitiligo repigmentation, and ask their patients to stay away from vitamin C supplements, and even ask their patients to limit the consumption of fresh fruits and vegetables that are rich in vitamin C.

Some patients did report that their conditions got worse after taking vitamin C, while others didn't notice any difference.

I barely took vitamin C supplement during the last two years of treatment, but I have been eating a variety of fruits (apples, oranges, grapes, kiwis, pears, watermelons, etc.) and drink orange and pineapple juice regularly without noticing any negative impact on my recovery.

MINERALS

Minerals, such as selenium, copper, zinc, and manganese, are the key components of antioxidant enzymes, which reduce the oxidative stress within our bodies. They also play critical roles in many biological processes. Calcium, another beneficial mineral element in vitiligo treatment, is closely related to the melanogenesis process.

Zinc

Zinc is critical to the melanin formation process and it can help repair vitiligo lesions. Many doctors believe taking zinc supplement is beneficial to vitiligo recovery and will prescribe it to their patients, especially during the active stage.

It has been reported that the combination of oral zinc and topical corticosteroids was more effective than topical corticosteroids alone in treating vitiligo.

Zinc can be found in a wide variety of foods. Oysters are considered the best source of zinc. Red meat, poultry, seafood, and fortified breakfast cereals are also good sources of zinc. In addition, various forms of zinc dietary supplements are available in the market.

Copper

Copper, like zinc and selenium, is associated with many life-supporting biochemical processes.

Some doctors consider copper to be a beneficial element to vitiligo treatment and encourage patients to take copper supplement or even use copperware to contain drinking water. However, there are opposite opinions from others who claimed that copper was irrelevant in vitiligo treatment.

This is likely an issue specific to each individual patient. Some people's vitiligo may have something to do with copper deficiency although this is not the case for others. If the blood test results reveal a low copper level, then copper supplements should be considered.

Calcium

Insufficient calcium uptake can affect the melanogenesis process. Several treatments, including the one using vitamin D derivatives, work by regaining calcium balance inside a patient's system, either directly or indirectly.

OTHER SUPPLEMENTS

Many other dietary supplements and medications have been proved effective in treating vitiligo.

Calcipotriol

Calcipotriol is a derivative of vitamin D, which is a hormone involved in mineral metabolism and bone growth. One of its important roles is to facilitate intestinal absorption of calcium. It has been reported that defective calcium uptake could inhibit the melanogenesis process.

Calcipotriol has been used to treat adult and child vitiligo patients with encouraging results, and is available as cream, gel, and ointment. Dovonex is a brand name calcipotriol ointment.

Ginkgo Biloba

As one of the most popular herb dietary supplements sold in the market, ginkgo biloba has antioxidant and immunomodulatory properties, in addition to its well-known memory and circulation enhancement functions. Although the exact mechanism of action is not known, ginkgo biloba is considered to have the potential of reducing oxidative stress, which is a possible cause for vitiligo.

Ginkgo biloba extract given orally has been reported to show positive outcomes in controlling the active progression of vitiligo and inducing repigmentation [9]. Several people have reported, through internet forums, that they had obtained repigmentation after taking ginkgo biloba.

It was also reported that the combination of ginkgo biloba with phototherapy (sunlight, NBUVB, excimer laser, etc.) was more effective than ginkgo biloba alone.

However, ginkgo biloba should be taken with some caution because it is anticoagulant and might cause internal bleeding for certain people. As recommended, ginkgo biloba should not be used by patients who have hemophilia or other bleeding disorders, or be taken concurrently with aspirin or other blood thinning medicines.

Fish Oil/Omega-3

Fish oil contains omega-3 fatty acids, which is beneficial to vitiligo treatment because it can inhibit inflammation and protect the body against autoimmunity. Fish oil also has many other health benefits.

Some vitiligo patients have reported positive results from taking fish oil. I have been taking fish oil on and off for a while for other reasons. The lesions appeared to be stabilized and shrinking slowly while I was taking it regularly, although I have not done anything to further verify the connection.

Considering the many health benefits of fish oil, it won't be a bad idea to consider adding it to your list of supplements.

St. John's Wort

St. John's Wort is an herb supplement commonly used for treating minor depression. Since it contains psoralen ingredient, some patients have used it as a photosensitizer, along with phototherapy, to treat vitiligo and reported encouraging results. Other items that also contain psoralen include figs, carrots, celery, parsley, grapefruit, lemons, and limes, etc.

CoQ10

CoQ10 (Coenzyme Q10) is an important enzyme and it can help convert food into energy within our bodies. CoQ10 is found in almost every cell in the body and is a powerful antioxidant. It can neutralize free radicals and may reduce or even help prevent some of the damage they cause.

Probiotics

A decrease in beneficial bacteria may lead to digestive tract disorders, which may prevent the body from absorbing needed nutrients and cause food sensitivity or allergy problems. Some digestive disorders might have connections with vitiligo.

Probiotics are good bacteria that help maintain a balanced environment in the intestines by restricting the growth of harmful bacteria. Probiotics may be used to treat many digestive disorders, such as diarrhea, gas, cramping, and infections, etc. They can also help regulate immune response.

L-Tyrosine

L-Tyrosine is an amino acid that is used to produce noradrenaline and dopamine, both of which stimulate alertness and increase energy.

Some patients reported that L-Tyrosine, along with high potency vitamin B, helped repigmentation. L-Tyrosine is available from drug stores as a dietary supplement.

L-Phenylalanine

L-Phenylalanine is a form of phenylalanine and an essential amino acid in the proteins. It is converted into L-Tyrosine inside human bodies.

The uptake and turnover of L-Phenylalanine in melanocytes is vital for the melanin producing process and is affected by calcium.

L-Phenylalanine can be taken orally, or be made into cream for topical use. Topical L-Phenylalanine cream with sunlight exposure has been reported to produce good results for some patients.

Major dietary sources of L-Phenylalanine include meat, fish, eggs, cheese, and milk. L-Phenylalanine is also available from drug stores as a dietary supplement.

Pseudocatalase

Catalase is an enzyme that brings about the decomposition of hydrogen peroxide into water and oxygen, and thus the reduction of oxidative stress.

Pseudocatalase is a compound that functions similarly to catalase. Researchers in Germany achieved encouraging results after treating patients with topical application of pseudocatalase and calcium, along with short-term UVB light exposure. Complete repigmentation on the faces and hands appeared in 90% of the group treated, and none of the patients treated developed new lesions or had any recurrence during a 2-year follow-up [3]. However, a few studies from other research groups failed to duplicate similar efficacy.

There are now two types of pseudocatalases available: PC-KUS and PCAT. At present, their availability in the US market might be limited.

Melagenina

Melagenina is a topical lotion manufactured in Cuba for treating vitiligo. It is an alcoholic extract from human placenta and contains placental lipoprotein fraction.

The placenta is an organ that has various essential nutrients and immune chemicals, such as hormones, proteins, lipids, nucleic acids, glycosaminoglycan, amino acids, vitamins, and various minerals. The placentas have long been used for treating health issues in many countries.

The latest version of this topical lotion is called Melagenina

Plus. There is some buzz on the internet about this lotion. Some people have claimed successful repigmentation after using Melagenina. I have not personally tried it, and just list it here for information only.

4. Treatments & Therapies

INTRODUCTION

Even though a universal cure is yet to be discovered, numerous treatments for vitiligo have been studied and used all over the world. New discoveries and progress are being made every year.

Today, a range of new and traditional therapies, which have brought improvement or even complete recovery to many vitiligo patients, are available. This chapter will briefly go over the common treatments for vitiligo. There are essentially two types of treatments for vitiligo: the ones that work from inside of our biological systems, and the ones that work from outside.

The external treatment options include various phototherapies and topical medications.

For phototherapies, first we have the free and natural sunlight; then there is the latest and the greatest 308-nm excimer laser, which is safe, effective, but relatively expensive; there is also the safe, effective, and affordable 311-nm NBUVB, which is now available for convenient home use.

For topical medications, tacrolimus and pimecrolimus have been used worldwide as the de facto standard topical medications for vitiligo because of their effectiveness and safety. Patients can also consider corticosteroids, photosensitizers and calcipotriol.

The internal treatment options include various oral medicines, dietary supplements and diet management.

Many of the highly effective solutions are in fact a combination of two of more treatments, which often includes UV phototherapy as one of the key components. The synergy of a combinational treatment often offers better results than a monotherapy.

For most people, vitiligo is the reflection of certain underlying health issues. Without properly addressing the internal causes of vitiligo, repigmentation through topical treatment alone might not be effective or sustainable, and relapse could happen. The ultimate solution should be treating vitiligo from both inside and outside.

Diet management can help us achieve a healthy and balanced system, therefore should be one of the focal points in a good vitiligo treatment solution. In fact, diet management has helped many patients achieve repigmentation and has been proved to be a natural, safe, and effective treatment that works from the inside.

There are many promising solutions for the vitiligo patients. If a patient stays positive and invests some time, efforts, and patience, he sure can find a solution that works best for him.

THE WALL STAIN ANALOGY

Imagine a water pipe inside a wall is leaking. The moisture gets on the drywall and causes mold to grow and stains to appear on the external surface. You can spray some bleach on the surface to get rid of the stains; you can repaint the wall to hide the stains; or you can even replace the drywall with a brand new piece.

However, as long as the leaking pipe is not properly fixed, the stains and mold are guaranteed to come back. The ultimate and sustainable solution would be fixing the leakage from inside, as well as removing the stains from outside.

The same principle applies in vitiligo treatment. Diet management and oral medication are the work done from inside, similar to fixing the leaking pipe. Topical medications and phototherapies are the repair work done to the outside, similar to removing the stains on the external surface.

DIET MANAGEMENT

"Let food be thy medicine and medicine be thy food" said ancient Greek physician Hippocrates

The outputs of our body, including our health, intelligence and physical appearance, are affected by the inputs, such as the food, air, drink, medication, as well as visual and audio stimulations.

The food and drink we consume every day are the essential factors that affect our health. Many cultures have a long history of treating health issues with diet therapy.

Medical researchers have discovered that cancer cells can be starved to death by controlling the patient's diet. Dr. William Li, president of the Angiogenesis Foundation, reported that eating the right food can prevent or fight off cancers through inhibiting excessive angiogenesis process, which grows new blood vessels that could feed the hidden or active cancer cells. Along with many other healthy eating suggestions, Dr. Li recommended chewing leafy greens to benefit from the enzymes, which are embedded deeply in the leaves and can activate cancer-fighting molecules.

From the experiences of many people who have achieved repigmentation, diet was a crucial factor in their recovery. Very likely, diet could have been one of the triggers for many people's vitiligo. It could also be the key factor that initiated and sustained many people's successful recovery.

Vitiligo is caused by certain issues inside our biological systems. It is the body's way of telling us something is not working properly and needs our attention. Topical medications and phototherapies repair the vitiligo lesions at the skin level. Without addressing the internal root causes, the repigmentation may not be effective or sustainable after the external treatment is discontinued. *Therefore, diet management can be of great importance in achieving successful and sustainable repigmentation.*

To me, the general principle of a healthy diet has two main parts: supplying the body with the nutrients needed and restricting the substances that are harmful.

Staying Alkaline

The human body needs to maintain appropriate pH settings to function properly. Here pH stands for the Power of Hydrogen and is used to measure the acidity and alkalinity of substances. It is a number between zero and 14: zero represents strong acidity; 14 represents strong alkalinity; and a pH value of seven represents a neutral and balanced state. Normally, the blood of a healthy human being should be slightly alkaline, with a pH value around 7.4.

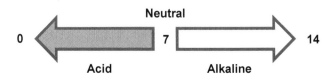

Many health problems originate from over acidity. In his book *Alkalize or Die*, Dr. Theodore A. Baroody stated: "The countless names of illnesses do not really matter. What does matter is that they all come from the same root cause...too much tissue acid waste in the body!"

We can shift away from excessive acidity by adjusting our diets: cutting down the consumption of highly acid items and eating more alkaline foods. Please be aware, the acidity of a food is not simply determined by its taste; rather, it is determined by the end products of its metabolism inside our bodies.

For example, lemons may taste sour, but they are in fact highly alkaline fruits. This is because lemons contain a lot of acid-neutralizing minerals, such as calcium, magnesium, potassium, and selenium; and the citric acid in them is weak. After metabolism, lemons' ultimate effect is alkalizing and will raise the pH value of the blood. On the other hand, some drinks might taste alkaline, but are actually highly acid.

Some vitiligo patients have reported successful repigmentation after drinking fresh spinach juice, or green juice that includes raw spinach and kale. It is noteworthy that raw spinach is a strong alkaline vegetable. However, cooked spinach is mild acid, so it is better to eat spinach fresh and raw.

A short list of alkaline and acid foods is provided below for reference. Readers are encouraged to learn more from various online sources.

Category	Alkaline Food	Acid Food
Fruits	Lemons, limes Watermelons Grapefruits Apples	Blackberries Cranberries Peanuts Plums
Vegetables	Asparagus Onions Raw spinach Broccoli Garlic	Potatoes Cooked spinach
Drink	Green tea Lemon water Soy milk	Milk Beer Coffee
Others	Olive oil Tofu Raw honey Raw sugar Flax seed oil Maple syrup	All meats White rice White flour Pasta Chocolate Cheese

Maintaining a Balanced and Healthy Diet

Many health issues start from an unhealthy and unbalanced diet. Please make sure your diet is well balanced to provide all the nutrients needed to support a healthy biological system.

For example, many vitiligo patients also suffer from deficiency of vitamin B12, folate, zinc, copper, or even vitamin C. Vitamin B12 deficiency could be an issue especially for strict vegetarians because natural vitamin B12 only exists in animal foods.

Vegetables rich in carotenoids, such as carrots, spinach, asparagus, and broccoli, are considered beneficial to vitiligo patients because they are excellent free radical removers.

Each individual may have his own specific nutrient needs to balance his system, but in general, food with sufficient antioxidants and various B vitamins are helpful for vitiligo patients.

Consider limiting your consumption of processed food and soft drinks, and eat more fresh fruits and vegetables, especially raw green leafy vegetables.

Sorting out the Foods that Disturb You

Certain foods can be one man's enjoyment and another man's poison. Some people are aware of the foods they have trouble with, either from past experience or through lab testing, but many do not know exactly what disturbs them. Very often, problems caused by foods would simply be dismissed as random incidents.

It is not easy to sort out the foods that cause trouble. It takes careful observation and analysis. An extensive allergy test may also help. The tricky part is, some foods cause problems right away, but many others kick in slowly over time.

I keep a daily log of what I ate and the issues I experienced on my smartphone. With this log, I was able to identify some of the items that caused my occasional abdominal pain and skin itchiness.

While eating a lot of fresh vegetables and fruits is a good thing, make sure you choose them carefully. Today, many fruits and vegetables are grown with heavy pesticides, growth hormones and synthetic fertilizers. Their taste, sizes, and ingredients have dramatically changed. To me, eating a small organically grown apple is healthier than eating a large one loaded with pesticides and growth hormones, even though they are all apples. Farmed shrimps, crawfish, and sea foods caught near the shore can also be contaminated with harmful chemicals.

I would avoid contamination in the foods by going organic as much as I could.

Some people believe that mango, red chili, cherry, raspberry, cranberry, and blackberry may aggravate vitiligo due to the plant phenol or tannins they contain. In my opinion, each individual might react to these items differently, but it won't hurt to keep an eye on them and see if they cause you any trouble.

Not Sure? Just Don't Eat It

With a variety of cuisines available in US, it is easy for someone to get enticed by certain exotic foods. When a person is healthy, his body is more compatible with and tolerant to various foods. However, the compatibility and tolerance would decrease if he is not in his best shape. For instance, a piece of medium rare steak and a few raw fish sushi are nutritious for a healthy person, but could adversely affect someone with an allergy or digestive issues.

There is no doubt that not all the foods are beneficial to vitiligo patients. Doctors practicing traditional eastern medicine would usually supply their patients with a long list of foods to avoid. Western medicine doctors, on the other hand, rarely put their patients on dietary restrictions.

It is a good idea for someone with vitiligo to be a little conservative and choose what he eats more carefully. If you have any doubt over the ingredients of an unfamiliar or exotic food, or your tolerance to it, just don't eat it.

Taking Care of the Digestive Disorders

Sometimes, it is not the food that causes problems; it is a person's digestive system that fails to do its job. For some individuals, medicines and nutrients don't work well because their digestive systems cannot absorb them. A compromised digestive system may also allow harmful substances to sneak into the bloodstream. If you have any issues with your digestive system, get them checked out. They might be the cause of other health concerns, including vitiligo.

Vitamin B Treatment

Vitamin treatment is a natural, safe and inexpensive therapy for vitiligo. It can be used along with other treatments such as phototherapy and topical medications. Its effectiveness may vary for different patients.

The Swedish Study

In 1997, medical researchers in Sweden published a paper titled *Improvement of vitiligo after oral treatment with vitamin B12 and folic acid and the importance of sun exposure* [1]. In a two-year study, Swedish professor Lennart Juhlin and his team treated 100 vitiligo patients with oral folic acid and vitamin B12, and requested patients to keep a record of sun exposure or UVB irradiation.

According to the report, clear repigmentation occurred in 52 patients, including 37 who exposed their skin to the sun in summer and six who used UVB lamps in winter. Repigmentation was most evident on sun-exposed areas. Total repigmentation was seen in six patients. The spread of vitiligo stopped in 64% of the patients after the treatment.

The study concluded that oral folic acid and vitamin B12 combined with sun exposure could induce better repigmentation than either the vitamins or the sun exposure alone.

Dosage

In the Swedish study, patents were given 5000 mcg (microgram) of folic acid and 1000 mcg of vitamin B12 twice a day. The total daily dosages were 10 mg (milligram) of folic acid and 2 mg of vitamin B12. These are quite high dosages compared to the recommended daily intakes for healthy people. However, vitamin B12 daily intake of 2000 mcg is not uncommon in medical treatment.

The Institute of Medicine did not establish any upper levels for vitamin B12 or folate (not folic acid) because of their low potential for toxicity, and no adverse effects have been associated with excess intake from food or supplements in healthy individuals. Yet high dosage of folic acid has raised some health concerns. Folate is considered safer for high dosage and long-term use. Please see chapter three for more details.

Patients who are interested in vitamin B treatment are advised to check with their doctors to make sure the dosages are appropriate for their specific physical conditions.

Safety

In this treatment, vitamin B12 and folate (or folic acid) should be taken together to be effective and safe. Taking folate or folic acid alone without vitamin B12 can mask the symptoms of a potential vitamin B12 deficiency and may delay the timely treatment of some serious diseases. Also, please be aware of the difference between folate and folic acid and choose the right supplements for your recovery.

TOPICAL CALCINEURIN INHIBITOR TREATMENT

Topical calcineurin inhibitors can be applied to the vitiligo lesions to suppress the local autoimmune activities and assist the growth and migration of melanocytes.

Medications

There are two commonly used medicines for this treatment: Protopic (tacrolimus) and Elidel (pimecrolimus).

Protopic and Elidel are both good options. Protopic appears to be more popular and better-known for vitiligo treatment. It is also considered more effective than Elidel. Please refer to chapter three and their respective drug information sheets for more details.

Usage

Protopic or Elidel are applied on the vitiligo lesions, usually twice a day. First, clean and dry the skin, then apply a thin layer on the lesions with your fingertip and massage a little. You only need to put on as little as possible because the skin is not capable of absorbing much. I personally use plain soap for face cleaning since I do not want to deal with the complicated ingredients in other facial cleansing products.

UV Exposure

Many medical studies have reported that Protopic or Elidel could deliver better and faster repigmentation if combined with UV phototherapy (natural sunlight, 311-nm NBUVB, or 308-nm excimer laser). One study even reported that tacrolimus would lack efficacy in the absence of UVB exposure [30].

However, there might be potential risks for such combinational therapies. More information on this topic is available in the later section of this chapter: The Power of Synergy.

Frequency

The cream or ointment is usually applied twice daily. The UV phototherapy, if used, is usually done 2-3 times a week.

Although some people reported repigmentation a couple weeks after using the treatment, usually it could take 2-3 months to see significant improvement for many others. Please stay patient, don't give up the treatment just because there is no sign of repigmentation after a few weeks.

Break Period

The medication guide for Protopic states: *Use PROTOPIC Ointment for short periods, and if needed, treatment may be repeated with breaks in between.* Similarly, the medication guide for Elidel also states: *Use ELIDEL Cream for short periods, and if needed, treatment may be repeated with breaks in between.*

However, no detail was provided on the implementation of the break periods. Patients are advised to consult with their doctors or the manufacturers on this matter.

Effectiveness

It has been reported that Protopic and Elidel appear to work better for lesions on certain areas (such as the face and neck), and might be less effective for lesions on the extremities or bony locations.

Risks

Topical calcineurin inhibitors (Protopic and Elidel) are relatively new drugs. Their short-term side effects include minor burning during the first few days of treatment, acne, and headache, etc. Their long-term side effects are not fully understood. In general, they are considered safer options than corticosteroids.

In 2005, the FDA issued a public health advisory on the possible cancer risks from using Protopic and Elidel. In 2006, the FDA required and approved updated labeling for these two medicines with boxed warning on the risks.

The FDA advised that these two medicines should be used only as labeled and not on children younger than 2 years of age.

However, the FDA also stated that a causal link had NOT been established between the medicines and cancers. In fact, the American Academy of Dermatology did not support, and many professionals in the medical community criticized the actions taken by the FDA and questioned the validity of the boxed warning.

So far, clinical data have failed to demonstrate a causal relationship between the use of these two medicines and cancers, especially for the Elidel (pimecrolimus) cream. According to one report [10], patients who used these medicines actually have similar or lower risks of cancer than the general population.

In fact, topical calcineurin inhibitors have been proved to be well tolerated and have good safety profiles during short-term and long-term use for up to one year with pimecrolimus and up to four years with tacrolimus [11].

Topical pimecrolimus and tacrolimus have been used to treat millions of people with atopic dermatitis. Pimecrolimus is primarily used for mild atopic dermatitis, while tacrolimus is commonly used for more severe cases. They both exhibit a more selective mechanism of action and do not affect center immune cells. Clinical data further suggested a greater skin selectivity and larger safety margin for topical pimecrolimus [12].

CORTICOSTEROID TREATMENT

Oral and topical corticosteroids have been used to treat vitiligo for decades. Corticosteroids are prescription medicines with high risks of side effects, and must be used under the guidance of a doctor.

Systemic (oral or injection) corticosteroids are the first-line treatment for patients with rapidly progressing vitiligo. It can stop the progression of the condition and also induce repigmentation.

Topical corticosteroids are applied directly to the vitiligo lesions to suppress the local immune activities. They are still being used by many doctors today.

Medications

Many topical corticosteroids can be used to treat vitiligo. Please refer to chapter three for more information. I personally have used triamcinolone acetonide, as well as clotrimazole & betamethasone dipropionate cream, but didn't see any improvement. To be fair, I have only used them for a short period of time and cannot judge their effectiveness.

UV Exposure

Some researchers reported that the efficacy of corticosteroids increased if combined with phototherapy. For example, the combination of excimer laser phototherapy with topical hydrocortisone 17-butyrate cream has been proved to be more efficacious in treating vitiligo lesions on the face and neck [13].

Risks

Corticosteroids can cause severe side effects, so their usage must be closely supervised by a doctor. A well-known sider effect with corticosteroids is skin atrophy, which is the irreversible thinning of the upper layers of skin. For this reason, high potency corticosteroids should not be used to treat vitiligo lesions on the face.

Generally speaking, corticosteroids should not be used for continuous treatment that lasts longer than two months.

PHOTOTHERAPY OVERVIEW

Phototherapy, also known as light therapy, has been used to treat skin diseases since ancient times. Today, it has become an important treatment option for vitiligo because of its high effectiveness, minor side effects and good tolerance.

Ultraviolet Rays

The light sources used for vitiligo phototherapy can be natural sunlight or artificial light. The therapeutic spectrum for vitiligo treatment belongs to the ultraviolet (UV) range. UV rays can inhibit T cell activities and promote melanocyte migration and melanin production.

Ultraviolet is the invisible light with shorter wavelengths (higher frequencies) than the visible violet light. It is further divided into three segments: UVA, UVB, and UVC. The wavelength range for each segment is defined as follows (nm stands for nanometer):

- UVA: 315nm-400nm
- UVB: 280nm-315nm
- UVC: 100nm-280nm

The sun actually generates UV radiation that covers all three segments and beyond. However, the UVC in sunlight can barely reach the surface of earth because it is blocked by the air and the ozone in the atmosphere; the ozone layer also absorbs much of the UVB. Therefore, the UV reaching the earth surface is mostly UVA, along with a small portion of UVB.

Most of the artificial therapeutic light sources currently used in vitiligo phototherapy fall under the UVB category, although UVA is still used in some traditional treatments.

Common UVB Light Sources

Sunlight is a free and natural UVB source. In addition, there are three types of artificial UVB light sources that are commonly used in vitiligo treatment. They include:

- 311-nm narrowband UVB (NBUVB)
- 308-nm Excimer Laser
- 308-nm Monochromic Excimer Light (MEL)

Among these light sources, the 311-nm NBUVB and the 308-nm excimer laser are the most popular and effective.

The 311-nm NBUVB therapeutic light sources are available as fluorescent tubes, which deliver the UVB light in a nondirectional and continuous form of radiation.

The 308-nm excimer laser is the latest phototherapeutic technology. The excimer laser is in fact a super-narrow-band UVB. It features selective treatment with its directional monochromic beam. The laser can precisely target an area but the coverage is limited. It is more effective and also more expensive.

It takes 30 seconds to a few minutes to treat one lesion with the NBUVB, but less than a second with the excimer laser. However, the excimer laser can only cover one small area at a time; whereas the NBUVB can cover a much larger area, depending on the light tubes used. With full length NBUVB tubes, it is possible to treat the whole body all at once.

The Mechanism of UVB Phototherapy

It is believed that UVB irradiation can modulate the immune response and induce the apoptosis (a self-destruction process) of the T cells. According to a study [14], both the 308-nm excimer laser and the 311-nm NBUVB can induce T cell apoptosis, but the excimer laser is more effective in doing so.

UVB can also stimulate melanocyte growth and migration, as well as melanin production.

Broadband vs. Narrowband

Originally, people used UVB light sources that radiate UV rays across the whole UVB spectrum for phototherapy. Such light sources are known as the broadband UVB devices, which can cause severe erythema or burning.

People later discovered that the effective therapeutic UV rays for psoriasis and vitiligo come from a small range of wavelengths (304 to 313 nm). The UVB radiation between 290 and 300 nm has no curing effects, instead it causes skin damage. Consequently, narrowband UVB light sources were designed and produced to address this issue.

With the NBUVB, the energy distribution is focused on the therapeutic wavelengths; the non-therapeutic wavelengths are minimized. This allows patients to receive effective therapy with minimum side effects. Studies have showed that NBUVB below the erythema-inducing dosage can still be effective. This makes it possible to shorten the exposure time and further reduce the side effects.

Common Phototherapies

At present, four phototherapy options are commonly available for vitiligo treatment. They are listed below by the order of popularity:
- 311-nm narrowband UVB (NBUVB)
- 308-nm Excimer Laser
- 308-nm Monochromic Excimer Light (MEL)
- PUVA (Psoralen + UVA)

The 311-nm narrowband UVB and the 308-nm excimer laser are now available in many dermatological clinics and hospitals.

The 308-nm MEL is not widely seen yet at the time of writing, but it may gain more popularity down the road.

PUVA combines systemic or topical psoralen with UVA phototherapy and is also called photo-chemotherapy. Personally, I would stay away from systemic PUVA unless advised otherwise by a competent dermatologist with good reasons.

311-nm NARROWBAND UVB PHOTOTHERAPY

The narrowband UVB (NBUVB) phototherapy uses artificial NBUVB light with a peak wavelength of 311 nm to treat vitiligo lesions. The 311-nm NBUVB is an effective, safe, and inexpensive (when used at home) phototherapy option.

Light Sources

In the past, a vitiligo patient had to visit a hospital or clinic to get NBUVB phototherapy. Nowadays, NBUVB therapeutic devices of different sizes are available for home use at a reasonable cost. There are full size NBUVB chambers for treating the whole body, and there are also compact handheld NBUVB devices for treating small lesions.

The NBUVB phototherapy for vitiligo usually lasts several months. If you are capable of following the proper safety guidelines and operational procedures, the best solution is to purchase your own NBUVB therapeutic device and do the phototherapy at home. This will save you a lot of money and tremendous amount of time.

In US, a prescription is required to order medical NBUVB phototherapy devices or replacement NBUVB light tubes for personal use. Some overseas companies also sell NBUVB devices online and ship them to international customers. When placing your order, make sure that you specify *311-nm narrowband UVB*. Broadband UVB light tubes are also available and look nearly identical, but those are not the best for vitiligo treatment.

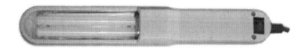

A 9W Handheld Narrowband UVB Device

The key component inside a NBUVB phototherapy device is the NBUVB tube. The majority of the light tubes used in the NBUVB phototherapy devices today are made by Philips. There are alternative NBUVB light tubes available at lower prices. However, according to a report [15], some of the alterative light tubes have different spectrum distribution, which outputs more power at the non-therapeutic wavelengths. Philips' NBUVB tubes have better quality and a longer history of successful clinic trials.

I would suggest ordering from a credible vendor and making sure that authentic Philips NBUVB tubes are used in their devices.

The NBUVB fluorescent tubes offered by Philips are designated by the /01 marking, while the broadband ones are marked by /12. For example, the 100W NBUVB tube from Philips is *TL 100W/01*, as shown below.

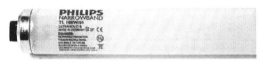

(Partial image)

Philips 100W NBUVB Tube: TL 100W/01

The picture below shows a Philips 9W NBUVB tube, which is commonly seen inside a handheld NBUVB phototherapeutic device. The part number is *PL-S 9W/01/2P*.

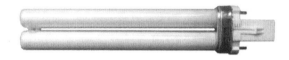

Philips 9W NBUVB Tube: PL-S 9W/01/2P

Choose a NBUVB device that is appropriate for the size and distribution of the lesions to be treated so the treatment can be done efficiently.

Just like regular lamps, NBUVB devices of the same wattage may come with different designs and packages. As long as the light tube used inside is of good quality, the design of a device can be of secondary importance. For instance, the embedded timer is not an important feature for me; rather it is another component that could fail. I have no problem using my smartphone as a timing device.

A well-designed device should have a reliable power circuitry and decent heat dissipation. For a Philips NBUVB tube, the radiant output decreases as the tube's wall temperature gets too high above the optimal 40°C.

Microphototherapy

There are also the so-called NBUVB microphototherapy systems, which can deliver directional NBUVB light to the targeted area using special optics, thus leaving the normal skin unaffected.

BIOSKIN, which is the NBUVB microphototherapy device offered by an Italian company, uses the Philips 311-nm NBUVB light tubes and can radiate a round light spot of one centimeter in diameter. Another advantage is that it only requires treatment once every 2~4 weeks according to the manufacturer. This sure saves the patients' time.

According to a study [16], 69% of the 734 patients treated with BIOSKIN for one year achieved excellent repigmentation (over 75% of the area obtained repigmentation), and 21% achieved good repigmentation (50-75% of the area got repigmentation).

However, such devices are expensive and heavy. They are only suitable for clinics or hospitals.

Dosage

Since the skin of each individual may respond to the NBUVB differently, treatment dosage is usually determined by experiments, especially for the treatments conducted at home. Patients can start with 30 seconds of exposure time, and then increase the exposure by 30 seconds in each of the following sessions until the formation of mild erythema, in which the treated lesion turns pinkish several (8~24) hours after the treatment. The dosage at this level is called the Minimum Erythema Dose (MED).

The initial treatment dosage can be 70~100% of the MED, depending on the area treated. For sensitive areas on the face, 70% of the MED is a good start.

As the skin becomes more tolerant to the NBUVB radiation over time, the dosage of successive sessions can be increased accordingly, usually by 10~20% for each session or each week. The exposure time should be reduced if significant erythema occurs.

The 311-nm NBUVB treatment is usually done 2~3 times a

week. Although it can be used during the active stage of vitiligo, the dosage should be kept well below the MED to avoid the Koebner phenomenon.

Operations

For new NBUVB tubes, Philips recommends a burn-in period of at least one hour to avoid the high initial output. Please follow this procedure whenever you start using a new replacement tube.

In order to get consistent results, a NBUVB phototherapy device should be turned on 30 seconds before the treatment. This is to warm up the tube and get its wall temperature to the optimal operating level. The tube will produce maximum radiant output at 40 C° wall temperature, but deliver only 60% of its maximum output if the tube wall temperature is only 20 C°.

Care should be taken to avoid direct NBUVB exposure to the eyes. Patients should wear UV protection eyewear while operating a NBUVB device. When treating lesions around the eyes, patients should keep their eyes closed and use UV blocking eye patches for extra protection whenever possible.

I would strongly recommend putting a warning label on the NBUVB device and keeping it away from the children! Also show the NBUVB device to everyone in your household and inform them of the potential risks so it wouldn't be used for unintended purposes.

Risks

The short-term side effects of the NBUVB include erythema and skin dryness. The maximum erythema would occur 8~24 hours after the therapy according to Philips.

As with natural sunlight, the long-term side effects of NBUVB might include the risk of skin cancer, conjunctivitis (snow blindness), and cataract of the eyes. However, no significant increase in the risk of developing squamous cell carcinoma or basal cell carcinoma has been associated with the long-term exposure to UVB. Both narrowband and broadband UVB have a significant lower risk compared to PUVA therapy. A study of patients exposed to UVB broadband or narrowband showed no significant increase in the risk of skin cancer [17] [18]. Other studies also concluded that NBUVB does not increase the cancer risks in any significant way and is safe to use [19] [20].

308-nm EXCIMER LASER PHOTOTHERAPY

Overview

In 1997, researchers in Hungary published a medical paper on treating psoriasis with the 308-nm excimer laser. The paper stated that the 308-nm excimer laser was more effective than NBUVB treatment. A few years later, the same team started treating vitiligo with the excimer laser. To date, researchers all over the world have studied the role of excimer laser in vitiligo treatment, and its efficacy and safety were well confirmed.

Today, the 308-nm excimer laser is considered the latest phototherapy technology in vitiligo treatment. It is a monochromatic and coherent light source, which can treat a specific lesion selectively while leaving the healthy skin unaffected.

Light Source

In 2000, PhotoMedex, a company based in Montgomeryville, Pennsylvania, received the FDA clearance for its XTRAC Lasers, which are now used worldwide in the treatment of psoriasis and vitiligo.

The XTRAC 308-nm excimer laser is generated by a xenon chloride molecular energy chamber. The Lasers can deliver a targeted, super-narrow UVB band to the affected areas.

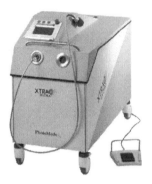

A 308-nm Excimer Laser Machine

Currently, there are several XTRAC Laser models in the market. Ultra and Ultra Plus are the two commonly seen models in various hospitals and clinics. Since these machines are very expensive and require special training to operate, they are not available for home use.

308-nm Monochromatic Excimer Light

The 308-nm monochromatic excimer light (MEL) source, which has the same wavelength as the 308-nm excimer laser but in a non-focused form, is also available. According a study conducted in France [21], the efficacy of the 308-nm monochromatic excimer light is similar to that of the 308-nm excimer laser. However, the excimer light would induce more erythema in order to get the same influence.

Dosage

The excimer laser is emitted through a small treatment head and can cover a small area (about 2cm x2cm for some models). The dosage, which is measured in mJ/cm^2, is determined by the doctors based on a patient's skin condition and tolerance. Patients usually receive 1~3 treatments per week.

Effectiveness

Studies have shown that the effectiveness of the 308-nm excimer laser treatment is closely related to the location of the lesions. It demonstrated higher effectiveness in treating lesions in the UV sensitive areas, such as the face, neck, and limbs. However, the effectiveness may decrease for lesions located on the UV resistant areas (bony locations, feet, and hands) [22]. Overall, excimer laser is more effective with localized and segmental vitiligo.

Safety

The 308-nm excimer laser is approved by the US FDA to use for psoriasis and vitiligo. In various studies, patients have shown good tolerance to the excimer laser phototherapy. It is a safe solution with a low risk of side effects. Most of the short-term side effects are limited to erythema and rare blistering.

The excimer laser can be used during the active stage of vitiligo thanks to its ability to suppress T cell activities.

Cost

Because of the expensive and sophisticated equipment, the excimer laser phototherapy is now typically available in hospitals and clinics and the treatment cost is relatively high.

Although each treatment session is quick and painless, patients will have to schedule time for the frequent trips to get the phototherapy, which is done 2~3 times a week and may last many months.

Limited by the small area of irradiation, excimer laser is more suitable for small and localized lesions, preferably less than 20% of the body surface area. Since the treatments are usually charged based on the size of the lesions, the expense can be quite high for patients with large areas of depigmentation.

PUVA

Overview

PUVA stands for Psoralen + UVA, which is a photo-chemotherapy combining topical or oral psoralen treatment with UVA phototherapy. PUVA was once the standard treatment for vitiligo; however, it has given away that position to the excimer laser and NBUVB due to its severe side effects.

Systemic PUVA

With systemic PUVA, patients are given psoralen (such as methoxsalen) pills or injections, and then exposed to UVA light. Systemic psoralen will cause the whole body to be photosensitive, so patients are required to wear skin and eye protections when going outdoors.

Systemic PUVA has significant side effects and limited effectiveness even after long-term treatment. Many patients may experience relapse after a year or two. This treatment shall only be performed by a qualified physician.

Topical PUVA

With topical PUVA, topical psoralen is applied on the vitiligo lesions, which is then treated with UVA. In a more general term, other topical photosensitizers such as Khellin can also be used, and UVA can be replaced with NBUVB or natural sunlight.

Topical psoralen only affects the area treated and has milder and limited side effects. It does not make the eyes photosensitive.

When using topical PUVA, make sure that the skin is not over exposed to UV light. Overexposure can cause skin damage and peeling, which may trigger the Koebner phenomenon and cause vitiligo to spread.

Risks

PUVA with oral medication has many side effects, including nausea, vomiting, dizziness, erythema, headache, and cataracts. Chronic and high dosage use of PUVA can increase the risk of skin cancers such as malignant melanoma.

Topical PUVA is safer, but can easily cause skin erythema and peeling if the lesions are overexposed to UV or sunlight.

Today, the excimer laser, NBUVB, and topical calcineurin inhibitors are better and safer treatment options for vitiligo patients than PUVA.

Alternatives

Other photosensitizers, such as Khellin, can also be used to treat vitiligo. Figs, celery, and carrots also contain psoralen. UVA can be substituted with sunlight, NBUVB, or excimer laser.

Khellin can be either taken orally or applied topically. Combinational treatment using topical Khellin and UVA usually takes a longer time to achieve repigmentation but also has fewer side effects. In general, Khellin is considered safe and effective. Even oral Khellin has only mild short-term side effects and few long-term side effects [23].

According to one report, topical Khellin 4% ointment in combination with monochrome excimer light has been used to treat vitiligo lesions on the face, neck, and knees, and it demonstrated much higher efficacy than phototherapy alone [24].

PUVA VS. NARROWBAND UVB

Researchers in England conducted a study comparing the efficacy of PUVA and NBUVB therapies [25]. A total of 50 non-segmental vitiligo patients were treated using PUVA or NBUVB, with 25 patients assigned to each therapy.

Their study showed that 64% in the NBUVB group, and 36% in the PUVA group, achieved good improvement (greater than 50% repigmentation). The color matching of the repigmented skin was also superior in the NBUVB group. It concluded that the NBUVB therapy was superior to the oral PUVA therapy in treating non-segmental vitiligo.

CLIMATOTHERAPY

Climatotherapy utilizes favorable climatic and environmental elements, which include air, temperature, humidity, barometric pressure, water, and sunlight, to assist patients' recovery from certain health conditions.

Among the various treatments involving climatic and environmental factors, Dead Sea climatotherapy is well known as an alternative treatment for many skin conditions, including eczema, acne, psoriasis, and vitiligo.

The Dead Sea is located in Mideast between Israel and Jordan. It is actually a salt lake about 1400 feet below sea level. The Dead Sea got its name because its water is nearly 10 times as salty as the ocean and no fish can survive in it.

The water there has a high mineral content and is considered by many to have therapeutic effects. The Dead Sea area also features amiable temperatures and sunny weather throughout the year. The air is rich with oxygen and low with allergens. Due to the low altitude level, the UV radiation from the sun is weakened and more suitable for skin treatment.

The therapy usually involves progressive daily sun exposure and bath in the Dead Sea, along with certain ointments, for several weeks.

SURGICAL SOLUTIONS

For patients who are not responding to the treatments discussed above, surgical solutions can be considered.

One of the popular vitiligo surgeries is epidermal grafting, which transplants a piece of good skin from a normal location to a vitiligo lesion to assist repigmentation.

Epidermal grafting is a quick way to obtain repigmentation and is an option for localized vitiligo lesions that have been stable for at least two years. It is crucial that the patients have been in the stable stage for an extended period of time, otherwise the repigmentation might not be successful.

SKIN CONCEALERS

It takes time for the vitiligo treatments to induce significant repigmentation. Before the skin completely recovers, cosmetic measures can be used to minimize the condition's impact on a patient's social life. One way is to use skin concealers to temporarily cover the lesions.

Some skin concealers work perfectly for dried skin, but can be washed off easily if you sweat or get wet. This is not a bad thing because that means they can be removed easily for topical medicines or phototherapy. However, they probably won't work if you are going to play golf in a very hot day.

More durable and longer lasting concealers are also available in the market, such as Covermark, and Dermablend, which can be water resistant if applied properly. These products offer different colors and shades to match a specific skin tone, so you will have to test them before making the purchase. Some products, such as Viticolor™ and Vitiligo Cover™, contain the sunless tanning agent DHA (dihydroxyacetone) and would last much longer. Vitiligo Cover™ contains both DHA and walnut shell and can last for days.

THE POWER OF SYNERGY: COMBINATION THERAPY

Overview

A lot of studies and research have discovered that the combination of two or more treatments, which usually include phototherapy, is more effective than a monotherapy.

For example, a treatment combining the Protopic 0.1% ointment with the excimer laser produces greater effectiveness and quicker response than the laser treatment alone. Topical corticosteroids, when combined with the excimer laser, also showed similar synergetic effects.

Several effective combinational therapies will be discussed below with references.

The Risks of Combinational Therapy

According to the manufacturer's instructions, UV exposure should be avoided while using Protopic or Elidel. This is due to the concern that UV might cause skin cancer when the immune system is suppressed. This is a valid concern, especially with systemic immunosuppressants. For Protopic and Elidel, which are used only topically, the long-term safety is not known and needs further evaluation.

Many researchers have done studies on the combination of topical calcineurin inhibitor and UV phototherapy. So far no severe side effect has been reported. In fact, one study reported that topical tacrolimus could actually protect the skin against UV-induced DNA damage in an experiments did on mouse skin [26]. A German research group reported that tacrolimus ointment didn't significantly interfere with the development or removal of local DNA damage in human skin [27]. Another study conducted by a Swiss group on human skin concluded that topical treatment with pimecrolimus or triamcinolone acetonide was not associated with increased epidermal DNA damage [28].

The conclusions of these studies are encouraging. Patients who are interested in these combinational therapies should get a better understanding of the risks involved and make educated decisions. The official opinions at the time of writing are as follows:

The long-term risks of combining Elidel or Protopic with UV phototherapy (such as excimer laser, NBUVB, and sunlight) are unknown, and such combinational treatments are considered as off-label use, which means they are not in accordance with the manufacturers' instructions. Patients considering such combinations are advised to consult their doctors and make educated decisions.

Vitamin B + Phototherapy

In the Swedish vitamin experiment [1], it was observed that the combination of vitamin B and phototherapy (with sunlight or UVB) could induce better and faster repigmentation than either the vitamins or the phototherapy alone.

Tacrolimus + Excimer Laser

It has long been noticed that vitiligo treatment with Protopic ointment works better in summer and on areas exposed to sunlight.

In a study conducted by French dermatologist Thierry Passeron and others [29], combinational treatment with Protopic and the excimer laser was compared with laser monotherapy. As they found out, the combinational treatment had excellent results (75% or more repigmentation rate) in 70% of the lesions treated, but with laser monotherapy only 20% achieved the same. For the UV-resistant areas, the difference is more remarkable: 60% of the lesions achieved excellent repigmentation with combinational treatment, and none (0%) of those treated with laser alone showed any repigmentation.

Even though the excimer laser is considered an advanced and effective treatment, it has limits as a monotherapy.

In another study where intra-individual left/right comparison was conducted [30], Dr. Passeron's group discovered that Protopic alone was less effective than the combinational treatment.

In conclusion, treatment combining Protopic and the excimer laser is much more effective than the excimer laser or Protopic alone.

Tacrolimus + NBUVB

In a study conducted by an Italian dermatologist group [31], the combination of tacrolimus ointment and NBUVB was used to treat patients.

According to the report, more than 70% of the lesions showed various degrees of repigmentation. About 42% of the lesions had more than 50% repigmentation. Lesions on the face, trunk, and limbs were more responsive to the treatment.

Pimecrolimus + NBUVB

In a study conducted by the Iranian dermatologists [32], the combination of pimecrolimus and NBUVB was compared with NBUVB monotherapy in a three-month experiment.

For the lesions on the face, the repigmentation rate with the combinational treatment was significantly higher than NBUVB alone (64.3% vs. 25.1%). However, there was no significant difference between the two treatments on lesions located in other areas of the body.

Corticosteroid + Excimer Laser

A trial was conducted by Italian medical researchers to compare the effectiveness of the 308-nm excimer laser with that of a combinational therapy, which involved hydrocortisone 17-butyrate cream (a topical corticosteroid) and the 308-nm excimer laser. The patients in the experiment have non-segmental vitiligo on the face and neck and previously were nonresponsive to NBUVB or topical corticosteroid treatment.

The combination therapy produced higher effectiveness than the excimer laser monotherapy [13]. With the combinational treatment, 21.4 % completely recovered (vs. 4.7% with the laser alone), and 42.8% achieved 75% or greater repigmentation (vs. 16.6% with the laser alone).

Calcipotriene + Excimer Laser

The combination of topical calcipotriene and excimer laser also delivers better results than a monotherapy. In a study [33] conducted in Tampa, Florida, three patients, who had extensive facial depigmentation and had failed to respond to a variety of topical treatments, all experienced 75% or more repigmentation after 10-20 weeks of combinational therapy, which included excimer laser treatment twice a week and daily calcipotriene application.

Dead Sea Climatotherapy + Pseudocatalase

In a study conducted by Dr. Karin Schallreuter and her group [34], the combination of Dead Sea climatotherapy and NBUVB activated pseudocatalase cream significantly speeded up the repigmentation than either therapy alone.

The study treated 59 patients who had vitiligo for an average of 17 years (range 3-53 years). Repigmentation was observed after 10~16 days with the combination of Dead Sea climatotherapy and pseudocatalase cream; usually it would take the conventional pseudocatalase monotherapy 8~14 weeks, or the Dead Sea climatotherapy 5~6 weeks respectively to achieve similar result.

REVIEW

After reading about all these medications and treatments for vitiligo, you might ask, "what should I do to get started?"

Very likely, you are going to need prescription medicines and a

UVB phototherapy device. Therefore, the first thing to do is to locate a friendly, competent, and open-minded dermatologist who is willing to work with you. Not every dermatologist has the right knowledge and attitude to deal with vitiligo; it might take some efforts to find one. I would say you will have a better chance by going to a clinic that is equipped with a 308-nm excimer laser machine or a 311-nm narrowband UVB chamber. The doctors there are probably more up to speed on vitiligo.

If your condition is in the active stage and spreading quickly, visit you dermatologist as soon as possible. You doctor will probably give you some oral immunosuppressants or immunomodulators to get the situation under control.

If you are in the stable stage, then you may consider diet management, dietary supplements, and topical medicines. Or simply ask your doctor what to do. Remember:

The successful and sustainable repigmentation for vitiligo should be achieved by addressing both the internal issues and the external symptoms.

Internal treatments, such as the diet management and oral medication, target the root causes of the condition; whereas external treatments, such as topical medication and phototherapy, target the symptoms and facilitate lesion repair.

Many patients have successfully recovered by addressing the internal issues through oral supplements, healthy diets, and healthy lifestyles. If your doctor only cares about the topical treatments, you will have to take care of internal part yourself. Review your diet, check out the B vitamins, make a plan, and execute it.

Among all the topical treatments, the 308-nm excimer laser, 311-nm NBUVB, Protopic, Elidel, and topical corticosteroids are all recognized as effective treatment options.

If money is no object and your schedule is flexible, the 308-nm excimer laser deserves primary consideration, especially for localized lesions. This treatment is safe, effective, quick, and painless.

If the lesions have covered a large area, then the 311-nm NBUVB phototherapy is more cost-effective and more convenient to use. Of course, it also works for small lesions and it is quite safe. The best part is you can buy your own device and do the phototherapy at home. You need no appointment, no driving, and no waiting; you can do it any time you want, and you will save a lot of money.

Protopic, Elidel, and various topical corticosteroids can be used with other treatment options to get better results. You would need advice and directions from your dermatologist on which one to use and how it should be used.

Don't consider PUVA unless you are out of options or your doctors thinks it is a good idea and has a good explanation.

Surgery is an option only if the lesions are not responding to medicines or phototherapies and the condition has been stable for more than two years.

As always, please consult a doctor for medical guidance and make informed decisions.

5. Personal Notes

Here are some of the ideas, thoughts and observations I documented during my treatment and recovery process. These personal experiences and opinions are presented here for reference only, and shall not be taken as medical advice.

MY TREATMENT REGIMEN

I used the combination of several treatments to heal my condition. The four key components are:

- Diet management
- Topical calcineurin inhibitor (Protopic and Elidel)
- UVB Phototherapy (sunlight and NBUVB)
- Dietary supplements

I also exercise a few times a week through playing tennis and golf. I occasionally practice meditation, which I believe is beneficial to my mind and body and should be done more often.

My diet management involved elimination and addition. I put several items, including shrimps, cabbage, and hot chili peppers, on my food blacklist. I also limited the consumption of seafood, canned food, non-organic meat, cheese, milk, and various berries. I started eating raw garlic and raw spinach regularly.

For supplements, I took 2000 mcg of vitamin B12, 2000 mcg of folate (folic acid in the beginning), and 1200 mg of fish oil daily.

In addition, I took 1 mg of probiotic, 50 mg of zinc, and 600 mg of calcium a couple times a week. I also took 2 mg of copper once in a while. Recently I started using a popular brand of calcium supplement that includes vitamin D3, zinc, copper, magnesium, and manganese. I tried ginkgo biloba briefly a few times but stopped doing so because I was not feeling well after taking it.

For topical medications, I used the Elidel 1% cream for about eight months, then switched to the Protopic 0.1% ointment. I used them on the lesions twice a day, once in the morning and once in the evening. I would wash my face with a plain soap, dry it with a towel, and then rub a small amount of medicine on the lesions with my fingertip. I usually put in a two-week break period after using Elidel or Protopic continuously for two months.

In the beginning, I used sunlight for phototherapy and would get 20~30 minutes of direct sunlight exposure in the mid-morning or afternoon.

Later, I started using a handheld 311-nm NBUVB light 2-3 times a week. I normally would use the NBUVB light after shower at night, but before applying the topical medicine. I also made adjustments to the frequency and exposure time based on the sun exposure I got during the week to avoid overexposure. I would only allow the lesions to get slightly pinkish, and I didn't increase the exposure time very often, usually once every two weeks.

KEEPING A TREATMENT LOG

It is beneficial to keep a detailed log on the treatment and recovering process. The log helps me keep track of the progress and identify things that might affect the skin condition. My log includes information such as:

- Medication and dosage
- Phototherapy duration and frequency
- Unusual food items
- Physical information (pain, itchiness, change in lesions, etc.)

I would usually write down short notes on my smartphone and then transfer them to a Word document once in a while. With the help of these notes, I was able to generate the treatment timeline chart in chapter one.

KEEPING A PICTURE RECORD

I would usually take pictures of the lesions at least once a week for record. These pictures allow me to go back and review how the lesions have changed overtime so I can evaluate the effectiveness of the treatments.

I tried to take these pictures from the same angle and at the same lighting conditions so it is easier to compare. I would also make sure the pictures were in focus.

Taking good pictures of the lesions on the face can sometimes be challenging because the skin on the face is highly reflective to natural light and camera flash. The flash often makes it difficult to see the details of the skin and should be used with caution. It is better to take the pictures with indirect natural lighting.

Regular digital cameras and high resolution smartphone cameras can both serve the purpose well. However, the front facing cameras on some smartphones may have very low resolutions, and are not suitable for this purpose. After taking a picture, always zoom in to see if it is in focus and make sure it provides sufficient details.

COMPARING DIFFERENT TREATMENTS

Since each person might respond differently to a particular treatment, you won't know which of the many treatments works best for you in the beginning. Doing some comparison experiments is the best way to find out the answer.

If there is more than one lesion in the same or similar areas, you can treat each lesion with a different option for a period of time. For instance, treat one lesion with corticosteroid and another with Protopic; or treat one side with Protopic and the other with NBUVB.

It is better to compare two lesions from similar areas. If you compare a smooth lesion on the nose with a hairy one on the chin, the skin difference might also influence the outcome. Obviously, this makes the conclusion of the experiment less convincing.

THE MAGIC OF THREE MONTHS

Three months seem to be a magical time span in vitiligo treatment. The three-month period was mentioned a lot as the minimum treatment duration in many medical studies and trials.

Interestingly enough, it took approximately three months for the lesions on my face to show significant improvement after using the Elidel cream.

This might have been a coincidence. However, the point is: vitiligo repigmentation is not an overnight process; it takes an extended period of time for some treatments to achieve noticeable improvement. If we are too quick to judge and give up prematurely, we might miss our chances for finding a solution.

Unless the side effects or the risks prevent me from continuing with a particular therapy, I would be patient and give it enough time before drawing a conclusion.

THE FOOD

I have suspected that my skin condition was a reflection of certain issues in my digestive system. These issues might have initially triggered the vitiligo and then certain foods made it worse. As part of my treatment plan, I made an effort to control what I ate. I think this effort has been critical to the recovery of my condition.

Shrimps

I used to eat shrimps regularly and really liked the flavor. However, it seemed that I would experience itchiness on the lesions, which would later get worse, after eating shrimps.

After some reading, I learned that shrimps could be highly contaminated, especially the farmed shrimps imported from some countries. Even for those caught in natural waters, contamination still exists due to the living environment and the habit of the shrimps. In traditional Chinese medicine, shrimps are considered as a prohibited food for people with skin diseases.

I decided this was not something I wanted to deal with. So I completely eliminate shrimps from my diet, and have not experienced any itchiness on my face thereafter.

Spicy Food

On two different occasions, my condition got worse after visiting my hometown for a few weeks. The purpose of the visits was to get away from my existing environmental factors (such as food, water, and stress) to see if my condition would improve. Apparently, something in my hometown had negative impact on my condition and made it worse.

It is a well-known fact that hot chili peppers are bad for many skin issues. I suspected the spicy food, which is a constant feature of the local cuisine, might have been one of the culprits. Therefore, I decided to quit eating very spicy items. With this change, I came back from a later visit to my hometown happily: the lesions didn't get worse this time; instead, it got smaller.

Vitamin C Rich Items

I regularly eat apples, bananas, oranges, watermelons, honeydews, and kiwis, etc. My favorite fruit is the organic mini gala apple. I also eat a lot of spinach, broccoli, celery, collar green, lettuce, and asparagus. None of these seemed to have any negative impact on my condition.

However, I barely eat berries, especially blueberries. They sometimes cause issues in my digestive system. And there is another good reason: most berries are acidic.

Raw Spinach

Several people have reported on the internet that drinking raw spinach juice or green juice with spinach in it had helped them achieve repigmentation.

Spinach contains numerous nutrients and is an excellent source of vitamin B, vitamin C, vitamin A, iron, magnesium, potassium, zinc, and copper. Spinach is also considered a good source of antioxidants because of the lutein and glutathione it supplies.

It is interesting that all these people reported using raw spinach. As discussed earlier, raw spinach is considered an alkaline food, whereas cooked spinach is slightly acidic. Eating raw spinach helps us stay alkaline and healthy. To avoid the harmful chemicals, I suggest choosing organic spinach whenever possible.

Raw Garlic

I have always suspected that my vitiligo has something to do with my digestive system issues, which had started almost a year before the initial depigmentation on my face. My suspicion is not groundless. It has been reported that digestive system disorders may cause the body's inability to absorb certain vitamins and minerals. The deficiency of certain important nutrients will eventually trigger health problems.

Inspired by the conversation with a doctor I met at a club, I started eating raw garlic regularly. After a week or so, the frequency of random abdominal pain and loose bowel movements decreased significantly.

Raw garlic is a highly alkaline food and a great source of antioxidants. It has many health benefits. For example, the anti-bacterial, anti-fungal, and anti-inflammatory properties of raw garlic can help a person restore the orders in his body, especially in the digestive tract. Garlic contains sulfuric compounds, which can reduce inflammation, and is beneficial for people who suffer from autoimmune disorders.

I usually take a clove of raw garlic during dinner or with some snacks because raw garlic can be very upsetting to the stomach if taken alone.

THE BREAK PERIOD

The medication guides for Protopic and Elidel recommend putting a break between short treatment periods, but provide no details on the specific implementation. Even though both medicines have good safety profile for short-term and long-term use, I still decided to put in the break periods.

I personally used a two-week break after two months of continuous Protopic or Elidel treatment. This may or may not be appropriate for other individuals, so please consult your doctor on this matter. During the break period, I continued using the NBUVB treatment and still noticed repigmentation, although at a seemingly slower rate, with the phototherapy alone.

NBUVB AND EYE PROTECTION

Please use extra caution when doing NBUVB phototherapy around the eyes, because UV rays can be quite harmful to the retina and the lenses.

I always wore the UV protection goggles when treating my neck with the NBUVB. However, the goggles would block the lesions near my nose when I was treating my face. I made two eye patches from a self-adhesive black felt sheet and used them instead. After a while, I realized that these eye patches were not completely blocking the light and I got concerned. I later switched to a solid black foam sheet that wouldn't let any light through.

I did some research and was relieved to know that the eyelids could actually protect our eyes from UV radiation. A study [35] conducted by researchers at Columbia-Presbyterian Medical Center in New York discovered that negligible quantities of UV radiation were transmitted through the eyelid skin, whereas 77% of the visible spectrum was able to go through. They concluded that using UV phototherapy on eyelids was safe.

Regardless, I still used my eye patches for extra protection when treating the lesions on my face.

THE ITCHINESS

It took me some time to realize that significant itchiness appeared to be a negative thing in vitiligo. In the beginning, I thought the itchiness was something random. After a few incidents, I noticed that the lesions would usually get worse after a surge of severe itchiness.

The itchiness on my face seemed to have something to do with the foods or the UV overexposure. Scratching seemed to make the lesions worse, so I later used ice to relieve the itchiness.

After I started the new combinational therapy, which involved diet management, vitamin B supplements, and Elidel cream, the itchiness never happened again.

HOMEMADE PSORALEN SOLUTION

Topical psoralen (or other photosensitizers) in combination with sunlight or UV phototherapy is a viable solution for those who have limited access to, or are unwilling to use, other treatments.

If you make your own psoralen solution with babchi seeds and alcohol, make sure to separate the seeds after the solution is ready for use in about 7~14 days. Otherwise, the solution will get more potent over time and may cause severe erythema.

When applying the solution to the lesions, first try it on a small area to get a feel and some experience. Usually, the solution should be applied lightly and sporadically to avoid sunburn. When exposing to sunlight or NBUVB, start from a short period of time and increase a little daily until you find the exposure time for minimum erythema (pinkish skin), which will only show up several hours after the UV exposure. Don't let the skin turn red or purple.

MAGNIFYING MIRROR

Feedback is important during vitiligo treatment, and I like to know how the lesions are improving. A magnifying mirror gives me the ability to see the subtle changes on the skin, and is a wonderful inspection tool for the lesions on the face.

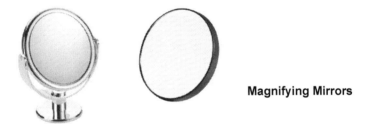

Magnifying Mirrors

Simple handheld magnifying mirrors with 5~12X magnification are available at supermarkets or department stores for several dollars each. I personally use a 10X mirror and it works great.

WOOD'S LAMP

A Wood's lamp is a skin inspection and diagnostic device. It is in fact a UVA fluorescent lamp with a radiant wavelength around 365 nm, nothing more complicated than the UV inspection lights that are used for checking passports and driver's licenses.

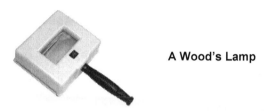

A Wood's Lamp

A Wood's lamp uses the fluorescence effect to enhance the contrast between a white vitiligo lesion and the normal skin, thus make it much easier to observe. This is especially useful in checking the early stage discoloration spots that might not be obvious under the normal lighting condition. A Wood's lamp can be purchased for 50~100 dollars.

6. Successful Cases

A lot of vitiligo patients have achieved remarkable improvement or even complete repigmentation through various therapies. During my research, I have come across many successful stories from various internet forums and support groups.

I picked some of the encouraging stories and put together a case summary for the readers. Only the cases that I considered credible were selected. None of these stories was associated with commercial incentives and many were supported by pictures.

I hope you find some of the treatments inspiring, and I also hope these stories can give you extra motivation and strength on the journey to your successful recovery.

The readers are advised to do their own research and consult their physicians before considering any of the treatments referenced here.

CASE 1: VITAMIN B + PROTOPIC + SUNLIGHT

A 25-year-old male had symmetrical vitiligo lesions on both sides of his face near the temple area. Each lesion was about the size of a quarter.

He achieved complete repigmentation on these lesions by combining oral medication, topical tacrolimus (Protopic), topical corticosteroid, and sunlight exposure. The lesions on his face started shrinking after two months into the therapy and completely cleared after four months or so.

Treatment

The patient was treated by a dermatologist and was prescribed both oral and topical medications.

His oral medicines included vitamin B12, folic acid, levamisole hydrochloride tablets, and thymopeptide enteric-coated capsules. He took these medications for about two months. The dosage was not reported. Levamisole is commonly used to eliminate intestinal parasites in human or domestic animals. In addition, it is also an immunostimulant approved for treating colon cancer.

His topical medicines included halometasone triclosan cream, which he used once daily in the mornings, and Protopic, which was used once daily at night.

Coincidentally, his job required frequent visits to outdoor construction sites, and he got plenty of sunlight exposure on his face during the treatment. In the pictures he shared, the recovering lesions appeared to be pink, indicating UV exposure.

CASE 2: VITAMINS + NBUVB

A young female at the age of 22 achieved over 90% repigmentation on the symmetrical lesions that almost completely covered her lower legs through oral supplements and NBUVB phototherapy.

Treatment

The patient took multiple oral supplements and used phototherapy for her lesions. She also contributed her recovery to eating an extremely healthy diet.

The oral supplements she took included vitamin B12, folic acid, grape seed extract, and calcium. Sometimes she also took vitamin D, vitamin E, magnesium, Omega 3, CoQ10, and flaxseed oil. She reported that the vitiligo stopped spreading after eating a healthy diet and taking vitamins regularly for one month. She did mention that she later had to take a break from the supplements because of nausea. Sometimes, mixing too many types of supplements could be an issue.

She used NBUVB lamps at home for her phototherapy and noticed brown freckles after regular NBUVB treatment for about three months. She believed that the NBUVB and the vitamins gave her the most significant improvement.

This young lady did not use any topical medicines on her legs. She had vitiligo on her face when she was much younger and those lesions were treated and cleared by using the fluocinolone acetonide cream.

CASE 3: SPINACH JUICE

A young female at her early 20s achieved complete repigmentation on the vitiligo lesions around her eyes by drinking homemade spinach juice.

Treatment

The patient achieved repigmentation after drinking two cups of homemade raw spinach juice daily. The size of the lesions was reduced by 50% after drinking the juice for about three months. She eventually achieved complete repigmentation with this natural treatment.

Her juice was made by mixing organic baby spinach, strawberry, honeydew, Greek yogurt, and water with a juicer.

CASE 4: GREEN JUICE

An adult male achieved repigmentation on his arms by drinking homemade green juice and eating a healthy diet.

Treatment

This gentleman contributed the repigmentation on his arms to the homemade green juice, which was made by mixing raw kale, raw baby spinach, bell pepper, ginger, celery, and apple using a juicer.

He also contributed his recovery to the change of lifestyle. He believed that reducing the stress level, staying happy and positive, and getting enough sleep had helped his recovery.

CASE 5: GINGKO BILOBA + COPPER

An adult female achieved repigmentation on the vitiligo lesions on her face and hands through natural supplements.

Treatment

The patient reported repigmentation on her face and hands after taking gingko biloba twice a day and wearing a magnetic solid copper bracelet.

The efficacy of Gingko biloba in vitiligo treatment has been confirmed by medical studies. Copper is considered by some doctors as a beneficial element in vitiligo treatment.

CASE 6: GINGKO BILOBA + SUNLIGHT + VITAMIN B12

A young male had multiple large lesions on his thigh. He had previously used the Protopic 0.1% ointment and the clobetasol propionate ointment 0.05%, which is a high potency corticosteroid, for two years with no success.

He later achieved repigmentation by using the combination of gingko biloba, sunlight and vitamin B12.

Treatment

The patient reported repigmentation on his lesions after using the combination of several treatments. He takes 120 mg of gingko biloba and gets 30 minutes of sunlight exposure on the lesions every day; in addition, he gets vitamin B12 shot once a month. He started seeing brown spots within the lesions after several weeks.

CASE 7: NBUVB

A teenage female achieved repigmentation on the vitiligo lesions on her hands and face through NBUVB phototherapy.

Treatment

The patient used NBUVB phototherapy and most of the lesions on her eyelids, forehead, chin, and cheeks achieved repigmentation after three months. The lesions on her hands and wrists also recovered, although at a slower rate.

CASE 8: PROTOPIC + NBUVB

An adult male achieved complete repigmentation on the vitiligo lesions on his face, neck and hand through the combination of Protopic and NBUVB phototherapy.

Treatment

The patient started with topical Protopic 0.1% ointment twice a day. He started seeing repigmentation on his hand after one month, but not on his face and neck. Later, he added NBUVB phototherapy to his treatment and achieved complete repigmentation after four months.

CASE 9: NATURAL PATH MEDICINE

A young female achieved repigmentation on the vitiligo lesions on her face through homeopathic medicine.

Treatment

The patient reported repigmentation on her face after resorting to homeopathic medicine after unsuccessful treatments by several dermatologists. Her lesions started to recover after she began taking medicines, which were not discussed in detail, to address the issues in her digestive system.

References

[1] Improvement of vitiligo after oral treatment with vitamin B12 and folic acid and the importance of sun exposure
Juhlin L, Olsson MJ.
Dept. of Dermatology, University Hospital, Uppsala, Sweden
Acta Derm Venereol. 1997 Nov; 77(6): 460-2.

[2] Melanocytes are not absent in lesional skin of long duration vitiligo.
Tobin DJ, Swanson NN, Pittelkow MR, Peters EM, Schallreuter KU.
Department of Biomedical Sciences, University of Bradford, Bradford, UK.
J Pathol. 2000 Aug; 191(4):407-16.

[3]Treatment of vitiligo with a topical application of pseudocatalase and calcium in combination with short-term UVB exposure: a case study on 33 patients.
Schallreuter KU, Wood JM, Lemke KR, Levenig C.
Department of Dermatology, University of Hamburg, Germany.
Dermatology. 1995;190(3):223-9.

[4] Successful Treatment of Vitiligo with 0.1% Tacrolimus Ointment
Lisa B. Travis, BS; Jeffrey M.Weinberg, MD; Nanette B. Silverberg
St Luke's-Roosevelt Hospital Center, New York, NY

[5] Tacrolimus ointment is more effective than pimecrolimus cream with a similar safety profile in the treatment of atopic dermatitis: results from 3 randomized, comparative studies.
Paller AS, Lebwohl M, Fleischer AB Jr, et al
Northwestern University Medical School / Children's Memorial Hospital,
J Am Acad Dermatol. 2005 May;52(5):810-22.

[6] Time-kinetic study of repigmentation in vitiligo patients by tacrolimus or pimecrolimus.
Lubaki LJ, Ghanem G, Vereecken P, Fouty E, Benammar L et. al
Dept. of Derm., Hôpital Erasme, Université Libre de Bruxelles, Belgium.
Arch Dermatol Res. 2010 Mar;302(2):131-7.

[7] Treatment of vitiligo with khellin and ultraviolet A
Ortel B, Tanew A, Hönigsmann H.
Department of Dermatology I, University of Vienna, Austria.
J Am Acad Dermatol. 1988 Apr;18(4 Pt 1):693-701.

[8] Long-term results in the treatment of vitiligo with oral khellin plus UVA.
Hofer A, Kerl H, Wolf P.
Department of Dermatology, University of Graz, Graz, Austria.
Eur J Dermatol. 2001 May-Jun;11(3):225-9.

[9] Effectiveness of oral Ginkgo biloba in treating limited, slowly spreading vitiligo.
Parsad D, Pandhi R, Juneja A.
Department of Dermatology, Postgraduate Institute of Medical Education and Research, Chandigarh, India
Clin Exp Dermatol. 2003 May; 28(3):285-7.

[10] Topical Calcineurin Inhibitors and Lymphoma Risk: Evidence Update with Implications for Daily Practice
Elaine C. Siegfried , Jennifer C. Jaworski , Adelaide A. Hebert
Am J Clin Dermatol (2013) 14:163–178

[11] Safety and efficacy of topical calcineurin inhibitors in the treatment of childhood atopic dermatitis.
Breuer K, Werfel T, Kapp A.
Department of Dermatology and Allergology, Hannover Medical University, Hannover, Germany
Am J Clin Dermatol. 2005;6(2):65-77.

[12] Immunomodulation and safety of topical calcineurin inhibitors for the treatment of atopic dermatitis.
Hultsch T, Kapp A, Spergel J.
Novartis Pharmaceuticals Corporation, East Hanover, NJ Dermatology 2005; 211 (2):174-87.

[13] Randomized controlled trial comparing the effectiveness of 308-nm excimer laser alone or in combination with topical hydrocortisone 17-butyrate cream in the treatment of vitiligo of the face and neck.
Sassi F, Cazzaniga S, Tessari G, Chatenoud L, Reseghetti A et. al
Centro Studi GISED, Ospedali, Riuniti, 24100 Bergamo, Italy.
Br J Dermatol. 2008 Nov;159(5):1186-91.

[14] Xenon chloride ultraviolet B laser is more effective in treating psoriasis and in inducing T cell apoptosis than narrow-band ultraviolet B
Zolta'n Nova'ka, Be'la Bo'nisa, Eszter Balta'sa, et. Al
J of Photochemistry and Photobiology B: Biology 67 (2002) 32–38

[15] New light source for narrowband UVB phototherapy puts patients at risk
Wiete Westerhof MD, PHD.
Color Foundation
Landsmeer, Netherlands

[16] Narrow-band UV-B micro-phototherapy: a new treatment for vitiligo
Menchini G, Tsoureli-Nikita E, Hercogova J
Dept. of Dermosciences, University of Florence, Florence, Italy
Journal of the European Academy of Dermatology and Venereology: JEADV 17:2 2003 Mar pg

[17] Light sources for phototherapy
Koninklijke Philips Electronics N.V.
Document number: 3222 635 49641

[18] No evidence for increased skin cancer risk in psoriasis patients treated with broadband or narrowband UVB phototherapy: a first retrospective study.
Weischer M, Blum A, Eberhard F, Röcken M, Berneburg M.
Acta Derm Venereol. 2004;84(5):370-4.

[19] No evidence for increased skin cancer risk in Koreans with skin phototypes III-V treated with narrowband UVB phototherapy.
Jo SJ, Kwon HH, Choi MR, Youn JI.
Acta Derm Venereol. 2011 Jan;91(1):40-3

[20] UVB phototherapy and skin cancer risk: a review of the literature.
Lee E, Koo J, Berger T.
Int J Dermatol. 2005 May;44(5):355-60.

[21] 308-nm excimer lamp vs. 308-nm excimer laser for treating vitiligo: a randomized study.
Le Duff F, Fontas E, Giacchero D, Sillard L, Passeron T. et.al
Department of Dermatology, University Hospital of Nice, France.
Br J Dermatol. 2010 Jul; 163(1):188-92.

[22] Treatment of vitlligo by 308-nm excimer laser: an evaluation of variables affecting treatment response
Ostovari N, Passeron T, Zakaria W, Fontas E, Larouy JC, Blot JF, et. al
Department of Dermatology, Hôpital de l'Archet 2, Nice, France.
Lasers Surg Med. 2004;35(2):152-6.

[23] Long-term results in the treatment of vitiligo with oral khellin plus UVA
Hofer A, Kerl H, Wolf P.
Dept. of Dermatology, University of Graz, Graz, Austria.
Eur J Dermatol. 2001 May-Jun; 11(3):225-9

[24] Monochromatic excimer light 308 nm in monotherapy and combined with topical khellin 4% in the treatment of vitiligo: a controlled study.
Saraceno R, Nisticò SP, Capriotti E, Chimenti S.
Dept. of Dermatology, University of Rome Tor Vergata, Rome, Italy
Dermatol Ther. 2009 Jul-Aug; 22(4):391-4.

[25] Randomized double-blind trial of treatment of vitiligo: efficacy of psoralen-UV-A therapy vs Narrowband-UV-B therapy.
Yones SS, Palmer RA, Garibaldinos TM, Hawk JL.
St John's Institute of Dermatology, Division of Genetics and Molecular Medicine, Guys, King's and St Thomas' School of Medicine, King's College, London SE1 7EH, England.
Arch Dermatol. 2007 May;143(5):578-84.

[26] Topical calcineurin inhibitors decrease the production of UVB-induced thymine dimers from hairless mouse epidermis.
Tran C, Lübbe J, Sorg O, Doelker L, Carraux P, Antille C, et. al
Dermatology. 2005;211(4):341-7.

[27] Tacrolimus ointment neither blocks ultraviolet B nor affects expression of thymine dimers and p53 in human skin.
Gambichler T, Schlaffke A, Tomi NS, Othlinghaus N, et. al
J Dermatol Sci. 2008 May; 50(2):115-22

[28] Production and clearance of cyclobutane dipyrimidine dimers in UV-irradiated skin pretreated with 1% pimecrolimus or 0.1% triamcinolone acetonide creams in normal and atopic patients.
Doelker I, Tran C, Gkomuuzus A, Grand D, Sorg O, Saurat JH,et. al
Exp Dermatol. 2006 May;15(5):342-6.

[29] Topical tacrolimus and the 308-nm excimer laser: a synergistic combination for the treatment of vitiligo
Passeron T, Ostovari N, Zakaria W, Fontas E, Larrouy JC, et. al
Department of Dermatology, Hôpital de l'Archet 2, Nice, France
Arch Dermatol. 2004 Sep; 140(9):1065-9.

[30] Lack of Efficacy of Tacrolimus in the Treatment of Vitiligo in the Absence of UV-B Exposure
Nima Ostovari, Thierry Passeron, Jean-Philippe Lacour, Jean-Paul et. al
Arch Dermatol. 2006;142(2): 243-253.

[31] Narrow-band UVB phototherapy combined with tacrolimus ointment in vitiligo: a review of 110 patients.
Fai D, Cassano N, Vena GA.
Phototherapy Unit, Dermatology Service, AUSL LE2, Gagliano del Capo-Maglie, Via Umberto I 16, 73052 Parabita (LE), Salento, Italy
J Eur Acad Dermatol Venereol. 2007 Aug;21(7):916-20.

[32] The efficacy of pimecrolimus 1% cream plus narrow-band ultraviolet B in the treatment of vitiligo: a double-blind, placebo-controlled clinical trial.
Esfandiarpour I, Ekhlasi A, Farajzadeh S, Shamsadini S.
Kerman Medical University, Dept. of Dermatology, Kerman, Iran.
J. Dermatolog Treat. 2009; 20(1):14-8.

[33] Rapid Response of Facial Vitiligo to 308-nm Excimer Laser and Topical Calcipotriene
John A. Mouzakis, MD, Stephanie Liu, MD, George Cohen, MD
J Clin Aesthet Dermatol. 2011 June; 4(6): 41–44.

[34] Rapid initiation of repigmentation in vitiligo with Dead Sea climatotherapy in combination with pseudocatalase (PC-KUS).
Schallreuter KU, Moore J, Behrens-Williams S, Panske A, Harari M.
Department of Biomedical Sciences, University of Bradford, UK.
Int J Dermatol. 2002 Aug;41(8):482-7.

[35] Present status of eyelid phototherapy. Clinical efficacy and transmittance of ultraviolet and visible radiation through human eyelids.
Prystowsky JH, Keen MS, Rabinowitz AD, Stevens AW, DeLeo VA.
Dept. of Dermatology, Columbia-Presbyterian Medical Center, New York
J Am Acad Dermatol. 1992 Apr;26(4):607-13.

ABOUT THE AUTHOR

Xichao Mo graduated with a master's degree in electrical engineering, and is now an electrical engineering and digital design consultant. He had previously worked as a senior hardware engineer and engineering leader at Hitech Electronic Displays, and then as a lead electrical engineer at GE Aviation.

Email: viti.help@gmail.com

Printed in Great Britain
by Amazon